PRAISE
THE CANCER

"Sarah McDonald is one of the most inspiring people I know. This book captures what I had the opportunity to see in person when I was CEO of eBay—how her authenticity, positive mindset and true courage helped transform everyone around her."

—John Donahoe, CEO of Nike

"The *Cancer Channel* offers us a front passenger seat on the journey to fight cancer. Whether you are battling it yourself, know someone who is, or want to read an incredible story of raw and real resilience—this book is for you."

—Kate Berardo, Vice President of Leader Development at Meta

"Sarah's memoir not only captures her powerful journey, lessons learned, and tremendous fortitude, but it is a strong call to action for employers everywhere to take a hard look at how they can better support their employees struggling with life-threatening diseases. She is living proof that providing the time and space to fully heal leads to better outcomes for the employee and greater loyalty to the company."

—Jennifer Brown, founder of Jennifer Brown Consulting, speaker, and author of *INCLUSION, How to be an inclusive Leader,* and *Beyond Diversity*

"Equal parts heartbreaking and hopeful, this is a wonderful story of perseverance amidst an improbable battle with not one but two cancers. Sarah brings this to life in a witty and engaging way that gives you real insight into what it is really like to go toe-to-toe with this terrible disease—and come out on the other side."

—Rob Fauber, President & Chief Executive Officer at Moody's Corporation

"This is the book you hope you or a loved one will never need to read. *The Cancer Channel* is Sarah's personal and unvarnished experience with the belief that cancer becomes less scary when we can talk openly about it. With humility and humor, she brilliantly shares her personal struggle to help bring hope and courage to anyone in their fight against cancer."

—Eric Ryan, co-founder of method and OLLY

"Not only does Sarah delve into the unknowns of a rare cancer diagnosis, but her journey resonates with every person impacted by cancer. It's a story about the fragility of life, human resilience, and the power of turning gratitude into action. We are grateful to Sarah reminding us that 'extraordinary moments do happen on ordinary days.'"

—Pascale Reich, president of Adenoid Cystic Carcinoma Organization International (ACCOI)

"I laughed. I cried. I couldn't sleep because I couldn't put the book down. Sarah's humanity and humor kept me talking about her story long after I put the book down."

—Amy Norman, founder and CEO of Little Passports

"This book is a window into the mind of a 40-year-old woman fighting two cancers simultaneously, while handling the pressures of a career and marriage. Not only does it include the elements of fear, bravery, and triumph you'd expect from a book like this, but it's also filled with a metrics-based process and humor that are unexpected and will make you laugh out loud."

—Rob Chesnut, former general counsel at Airbnb and author of the bestselling book *Intentional Integrity: How Smart Companies Can Lead An Ethical Revolution*

"Visceral, hilarious, devastating, and hopeful, Sarah McDonald has opened an intimate window to the lived experience of cancer and survivorship. I'd recommend this read to anyone in health care to remember why we do the work. I am a better clinician for it."

—Lyra B. Olson, PhD, Doctor of Pharmacology and Cancer Biology

THE
CANCER
CHANNEL

One year.
Two cancers.
Three miracles.

Sarah E. McDonald

ISBN: 978-1-958777-00-8 (paperback)
ISBN: 978-1-958777-01-5 (eBook)

Library of Congress Control Number: 2022912957

Printed in Mill Valley, CA USA by Sarah E. McDonald.

The author has strived to be as accurate and complete as possible in the creation of this book.

This book is not intended for use as a source of health, medical, legal, or financial advice. All readers are advised to seek the services of competent professionals in the health, medical, legal, and financial fields.

The advice and strategies found within may not be suitable for every situation. This work is sold with the understanding that neither the author nor the publisher is held responsible for the results accrued from the advice in this book.

While all attempts have been made to verify information provided for this publication, the publisher assumes no responsibility for errors, omissions, or contrary interpretation of the subject matter herein.

For more information, visit www.TheCancerChannelBook.com

For bulk book orders, contact: orders@TheCancerChannelBook.com

To Ruth and Kristin for being lifelines on Cancer Island

To Geoff for being everything I needed

To Rory for being

TABLE OF CONTENTS

Foreword   xi

Prologue   xv

Chapter 1: The Cancer Channel   1

Chapter 2: Wingwoman   11

Chapter 3: Wait. I Have Cancer?   21

Chapter 4: "Processing" My Cancer Diagnosis   29

Chapter 5: Are You Kidding Me!? Who Gets Two Cancers!?   41

Chapter 6: The Cancer Bombshell   57

Chapter 7: "Scanxiety"   71

Chapter 8: And So It Begins   79

Chapter 9: Preparing For Bald   89

Chapter 10: Lite Bright: Adventures In Radiation Therapy   101

Chapter 11: Mouth Sores Are Stupid And They Suck   113

Chapter 12: The F**King Goiter (TFG)   123

Chapter 13: Team Two   137

Chapter 14: We Make The Best Decisions We Can   147

Chapter 15: The Roller Coaster That Is Cancer   163

Chapter 16: Speaking of Cancer...   177

Chapter 17: Living With Cancer   191

Chapter 18: We Must Do What Is In Our Hearts   209

Postscript   217

FREE Gifts From Sarah!   221

Thank Yous   223

About The Author   225

FOREWORD

Leaders are used to surprises and plan for them. There are still some things you never expect. When Sarah came into my office and said "I have cancer," I knew we'd find a way to support her, but no one at the company was prepared for what that would mean. This book would have helped.

Shortly after moving my family across the country from New York to California to become President of eBay, Inc., I met Sarah to discuss the role of Chief of Staff. A good Chief of Staff can help a leader make a management team more effective by ensuring the agenda is the right one, meetings are high quality, and the team follows through. Hiring this role was a priority for me as I landed at the company in the fall of 2011.

I vividly recall our first meeting in a small conference room in eBay's San Jose headquarters. Sarah radiated warmth and energy. I could tell immediately that she was a rare combination of humanity, passion, and strong executive skills. She was perfect for the position, and accepted the role a few days later.

In the months that followed, Sarah and our team were exceptionally busy setting the agenda and the "operating rhythm" of the business. She wanted to help me understand the heart and soul of the business and the eBay seller community. We crisscrossed the country together for customer events. I soon learned that attending a seller meeting with Sarah is equivalent to being chaperoned by the Queen. Everyone loved her. Her influence on me was immense. She grounded me in the business. Her wealth of experience and vast network of employees, customers, and community drivers massively shortened my learning curve.

During these trips, I got to know Sarah beyond the job. She told me about her desire to have a child, about her struggle with infertility, and about her close relationship with her husband, Geoff. I became vested in her success as an executive and as a friend. She was loyal, hardworking, and effective, but most of all I realized that she was a great person.

She pulled me into a room during the winter of 2012 to confide she had a rare cancer. I was stunned. It was a gut punch to see someone like her going through one of life's worst experiences at such a young age. I really didn't know how to respond, but my first instinct was to make sure that she prioritized her health over work. I told her that she should immediately take paid leave. She left the office that day to begin her treatment program. The news shook our management team, but we vowed to do whatever we could to help her.

Over the next year, I kept in touch with Sarah, who would fill me in on her journey. At some point during that year, Sarah's updates went from discouraging, to mixed, to hopeful, to positive. Given the odds that she was facing, I approached the news of her early remission with cautious encouragement.

Three years later, when she told me she was in full-blown remission, I found it remarkable. Her success in getting pregnant with her daughter Rory after that seemed nothing short of a miracle.

When I read the manuscript for *The Cancer Channel*, it was an emotional experience. I thought I knew Sarah's story, but in truth, I had no idea of the hell that she went through. This no holds barred account is bracing, but it is also optimistic and even humorous in classic Sarah style.

Sarah's story is an invaluable resource for anyone touched by this awful disease. It provides a detailed view of treatment without sugar coating. If I, or a loved one, were going through something similar, I would want the unvarnished truth about the cancer journey. But, I would also want hope. I would want to know that the fight is worth it, and that no matter the odds there can be positive, wonderful, even miraculous outcomes. This account is a testament to the fact that relentless focus and positive will can deliver that result.

The Cancer Channel is also an important resource for companies considering policies for employees dealing with health issues. When we told Sarah that the company would take care of things, we were simply trying to help a colleague and a friend who was facing a crisis. We did not fully understand all of the implications for the business. What happened was that her recovery would become a source of inspiration for everyone in our company, and a point of pride for our culture. Now Sarah's story can go on to inspire others and maybe make them feel not so alone in the most alone of times.

Devin Wenig, founder and principal, Norse Capital;
Former CEO of eBay, Inc.

PROLOGUE

"Mommy. I keep all of my magic in my heart. Is that where you keep yours?"

I am sitting with my girl across my lap on the dense, cozy rug in front of our couch. It is mid-afternoon and I have picked her up early from her after school program so that she can have the just-Mommy-and-Rory time she had asked for this morning on our drive to school. She is now big enough that really only her head and her torso can rest on what she calls my "special place" – my lap. "Mommy. Let me sit in your special place," she demands when we watch movies, when we are at dinner at friends' houses, when she needs a little reassurance or to feel like my baby again. Sometimes, when I need her to feel like my baby again, I'll pull her over to my lap – her long, gangly, six-year-old legs splayed out beside us. Those legs won't fit as I lean over to grab and hold all the parts of her I can still gather in my arms as I cover her face with kisses.

Twenty minutes earlier, this same yummy girl had been standing in front of me with crossed arms and a scowl on her face. She was demanding a ramekin of Cheez-Its® before she was forced to eat the healthy strawberries I had just cut up for her and she had stamped her foot to punctuate each word.

"We always eat a healthy snack first, Rory," I remind my stomping girl. "And I would love to hear you ask me kindly for the Cheez-Its® rather than yelling at me," I say, trying to maintain an even voice.

"I! AM! ASKING! KINDLY!" she screeches before sticking her fingers in her ears to block out anything else I might say.

I have been reading all of the child-rearing blogs and books recommended to me while Geoff and I both try to lovingly ride out the roller coaster of BIG feelings that is six. Dr. Laura instructs me that the child acts out because she feels disconnected from me. What I need to do is "establish connection" with her and the grumpy little troll standing in front of me will transform into the love bug I know she can be.

I ask if I can give her a hug. I receive a resounding "No!" and a half-hearted push. After several more attempts and more screeching, my girl finally gives in and lets me hold her. We slowly slump onto the floor and into a tangle of arms and legs.

I rock back and forth with my girl on the rug. She is now cooing at me and making baby sounds. The sun is streaming into our living room and we are bathed in its light. It is one of those enchanted moments in parenting when the world slows for you and your child and you are simply, utterly in love with this small human and her wondrous being.

"Mommy. I keep all of my magic in my heart. Is that where you keep yours?"

I cannot believe this beautiful thing she has just uttered. Truly, she is magical. I am so very lucky, I tell myself for the umpteenth time.

It might not have been like this. In one alternate reality, I was unable to conceive a child. In another alternate reality, I had never married. And in those infinite other realities, there had been the very real possibility that I wasn't going to – and didn't – survive my battle with cancer.

In 2012, I was a newly married, forty-something, tech executive undergoing fertility treatments when I was diagnosed with two unrelated, or *primary source,* types of cancer. "Primary source" means each originated at its own site in my body and was not a spread (metastasis) of the other. Each cancer was intent on, and capable of, killing me on its very own. My prognosis was unclear and I was told that carrying a child was off the table. I felt as if everything in my life had suddenly been taken away from me.

Over the course of one year, I underwent chemo, radiation, and multiple surgeries. I lost my hair and my sense of taste. But against what felt often like impossible odds of cancer statistics – I survived. And later, I carried a baby. My life that had been lost amidst those alternate realities was once again found. Who could have imagined it would be like this?

The concept for this book started with the blog I wrote during that year. I loved writing the blog. It allowed me to explore the sometimes ridiculous stories of physical indignities and personal struggle that a year of fighting cancer brings. And while I certainly experienced terror and pain that year, I also found a whole bunch of stuff to laugh about. In the end, finding the humor in my physical indignities actually helped me get through the larger experience.

I've read a number of cancer memoirs, beautifully written with clarity driven by the knowledge that life is precious and short; perhaps the most touching ones published posthumously. I loved diving into their stories and reading the visceral descriptions of the terror they felt (that *I* felt) when they learned they had cancer. Our shared experience made me feel less alone. But what was missing from these stories is the humor I found from the physical indignities of cancer treatment – the absolute ridiculousness you are (read: I was) willing to endure to claw your life back. I decided I needed to add my stories of hope, humility, and yes, humor to the mix. If my stories can help others who are finding their way on their cancer journey maybe laugh, then the ten (what?!?) years spent writing these stories down will have been worth it.

Since my diagnoses my husband Geoff and I have taken a very open approach to discussing my cancer – not hesitating to share my stories in detail if people are newly diagnosed or simply curious. It is our opinion that cancer (and even death) becomes less scary when we can talk openly about it. That said, Geoff and I haven't known exactly when it was "appropriate" to share with a child that her Mommy had cancer. She knows her grandfather died from cancer. One warm Saturday afternoon we had friends over for cocktails and these dear friends asked about my cancer status (as loving friends regularly do) within earshot of Rory. Rory perked up and rushed over to me.

"Mommy. You had cancer?" Her little eyes searched mine as I thought about how I would answer this question. I wrapped my arms around my little human.

"Yes, sweetie. I did. But the doctors used medicine to make me better and I don't have cancer any longer. You don't need to worry."

"Ok, Mommy – but I'm keeping my eye on you so you don't die! *And I mean BOTH eyes, Mommy!*"

CHAPTER ONE

THE CANCER CHANNEL

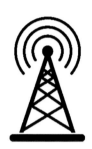

When I was first diagnosed, cancer (and dying) was all I could think about. There was nothing I could do—no conversation I could have, no article I could read—that wasn't interrupted by the relentless drumbeat in my head: *I have cancer. I have cancer. I have cancer.* And it really took everything I had within me not to voice that drumbeat and scream it aloud—to family, to friends, to the person checking me out at Trader Joe's. I called it the Cancer Channel, and its official slogan was, *"All cancer, all the time."*

My cancer diagnosis had horrendous timing (as if a cancer diagnosis could have good timing). I lived in the city I loved. I had just married a wonderful man, Geoff, with whom I was thrilled to be pursuing "happily ever after." I had just been promoted into a job that could transform my career. I felt surrounded by, and in steady touch with, many close friends. Most nights Geoff and I would turn off the lights and say "lucky us" to one another as we drifted off to sleep. Because we were lucky. Because we *are* lucky.

With my diagnosis, it felt like everything that had been falling into place was now simply falling. Everything I had worked for and hoped for felt like it was being taken away from me. I could no longer count on reliable truths I had counted on before—like *not* dying. Suddenly, my world went from sunny, saturated Technicolor hues to Cold War-era black and white. I lived in the middle of this bumping, colorful city that I loved to walk in – but now as I trudged, zombie-like, through my neighborhood, the colors were muted. Sounds were muffled by the refrain in my mind: *I have cancer. I have cancer. I have cancer.* How could others laugh and shout on the street, unaware that their lives could change in an instant by three simple words?

I believe all cancer journeys are unique and complicated and scary and often very, very lonely. Mine is no exception.

For me to tell it right, I need to rewind the tape to October 2004. I was single and living in a one-bedroom apartment in San Francisco's Fillmore district. eBay had just hired me as a global policy manager in a department called "Trust and Safety." The name had a Hall-of-Justice ring to it, like the team should be a bunch of superheroes with rare but totally *rad* superpowers.

But in truth, we were a bunch of MBAs who had been hired to create (and enforce!) the rules by which buyers and sellers would trade on the eBay platform. It was still relatively early days for ecommerce, and it felt like we were creating rules and writing policy where none had existed before—because we were. My workday felt creative and playful, like some kind of new frontier. It was a most excellent job.

I was full of hope and promise in this new role and so I also re-committed myself to my workout regimen. eBay had a gym and a salad bar, and I was determined to become a regular at both. After a month or so, I was pleased to see my weight was dropping and I was firming up. The not-so-great thing though was with the weight loss I also began to notice a lump in my left breast. Facing the mirror, I could see its worrying outline in the upper-left quadrant, nearest my armpit.

In October 2004, I made an appointment to see my new obstetrician-gynecologist, or OB-GYN. (Note: I am going to change this doctor's name to the very descript "Dr. ObGyn" and will use equally obvious – hopefully clever – monikers to help keep all of the doctors straight and their privacy protected). Since I had only been in San Francisco a year, I didn't really have a relationship with Dr. ObGyn. I liked her a ton though. She was about my age, wore hip, cool clothes, and had mentored my brother's friend through his residency.

What I remember most from this first appointment was my concern that I was making too much of this lump; I was wasting the doctor's time, I was being a hypochondriac. Dr. ObGyn felt the lump, agreed she felt *something*, and said she would recommend a mammogram even though I was only thirty-six. We had a conversation about how most lumps are simply fibrous masses, and so it seemed reasonable that this was what it was.

THE MAMMOGRAM

The imaging center didn't have an appointment for a couple of weeks. Since I was new to my job at eBay, I got the first mammogram appointment of the day at 8:00 am to minimize time off work. It wasn't supposed to take more than thirty minutes.

I am someone who likes to be efficient, so I scheduled an appointment with my (also new) general practitioner, Dr. Internist, at 9:00 am. With a comfortable buffer between appointments in the same building, I told myself I should finish by 10:00 am and, with the hour-long drive from San Francisco to San Jose, get to work by 11:00 am.

It was my first-ever mammogram, so everything was new to me. I arrived fifteen minutes early as instructed to fill out the medical history paperwork. I sat in a pleather turquoise chair in the waiting room. It was 2004, so I had no smartphone to occupy me while I waited for my name to be called. Instead, I had brought a copy of *The Economist* to keep my mind occupied. I think I know why doctor's offices have copies of *People* magazine instead of *The Economist*; the former distracts, the latter does not.

I was introduced to the realities (read: indignities) of modern medical technology with this first mammogram. Each breast is squeezed between cold plates as the patient holds her breath (and self-consciously sucks in her belly). I now understood why women had intimated that mammograms were something to be endured.

Once we were finished with the four x-rays (two of each breast), the technician sent me to the waiting room while she examined the results. Other women had arrived and they were reading *People* and other variety magazines. I decided to give in to this guilty pleasure and traded *The Economist* for a copy of *People* as I waited for the technician to confirm the images were okay.

After about 15 minutes, the technician returned and asked me to join her in the room again.

Huh.

She explained to me that she wanted to take a few more photos, which she did before sending me back to the reception area. More waiting. Less article reading this time. The technician returned and asked that I follow her...*again*. I asked her whether the (worrying) lump that had sent me to the OB-GYN in the first place was concerning her. She told me no. She explained that she had seen some "calcifications" on my images and sometimes doctors wanted extra photos of those. We took more photos. I went back to the waiting room.

At this point there was no way I was going to get anything read. I got to thinking about how I had brought all this worry on myself. *I* was the one who had talked the doctor into a mammogram. And now it wasn't even the lump that the technician was worried about. What were "calcifications," and why didn't I know anything about them? Why were they *concerning* to the technician? I thought about how young I was. I looked at the other women in the room, most of whom were older than my mother.

I listened as two of these women complained about their annual mammograms. They recited the indignities and discomforts of what I had just experienced. They grumbled about the hassle of setting up the appointments in their busy lives and expressed their annoyance that there was now a delay as the technician was running behind. "How could a doctor's office get so far behind this early in the morning?" they asked one another.

Part of me wanted to apologize to these women for messing up the schedule. Part of me felt very inconsiderate for making them late. But another part of me wanted to scream at them, "Don't you see that I've been called back three times now? Don't you think that's because there is a *problem*?! Don't you see that I am thirty-six years old and shouldn't even *be* here!?!"

The technician took 23 images in all.

The steady beat of *I have cancer I have cancer, I have cancer* began as my head started to tune into what I would come to know as the cancer channel. Gone was my concern that a mammogram might be painful. Gone was my concern about whether my belly looked fat. Now I just wanted the mammogram to be truthful. I wanted it to tell the technician and the doctors (and myself) that I couldn't possibly have breast cancer.

THE SONOGRAM
The technician returned and asked if she could do a sonogram to get a better look at the calcifications. I was led into another sterile, cold room. For the sonogram, they asked that I lay down on a table on my side with

a triangle-shaped pillow wedged behind me. The technician squirted some warm (*thank God!*) lubricant on my breast and used the sonogram wand to search on my skin surface for the calcifications that were lurking below.

The sonogram screen seemed to play a kind of underwater movie of my breast. Unfortunately, I had no idea how to interpret the images, so I started asking questions. The technician then explained sonograms can sometimes see things better than mammograms. She hoped the sonogram would allow her to view the shape of the calcifications, as abnormally-shaped calcifications can sometimes be an indication that there is cancer. *Cancer?*

The sonogram technician took images of my calcifications and assured me she would send them to Dr. ObGyn, who would call me to discuss what we should do next.

THE INTERNIST

I walked out of the imaging clinic and took the elevator to my Internist appointment. I was so distracted by all of the additional imaging that I hadn't thought to alert my Internist's office when my mammogram ran late—and frankly, I assumed (wrongly) the clinic and the Internist office would be in contact. Since I was now two hours late for my 9 am appointment, I waited an hour before they could fit me in. While I sat in the waiting room this time, I didn't read articles. I just sat and tried not to panic.

Once I was called back, I waited another hour to meet with the doctor. Beyond my concern with calcifications, I was now super anxious that it was 1 pm and I still had an hour's drive to get to work. I didn't have my new manager's mobile number, so I had no idea how to contact him to let him know where I was or how late I was going to be. And how was I going to explain to him what was going on? The later it got, the more anxious I became.

When Dr. Internist finally entered the room, it was clear she was worked up as well. She introduced herself and then informed me that by missing her first appointment of the day, I had derailed the rest of her schedule, and that being so late to future appointments could lead to dismissal as a patient. I was taken aback by her reprimand and quietly told her I'd spent the morning in the imaging clinic because they had found something. Because they thought I had breast cancer. "Oh," she said.

I started to cry.

I arrived at work at 3:00 pm. eBay didn't have a big work-from-home culture at the time and I felt a need to show up at the office to assure my manager I hadn't been playing hooky. I apologized that the doctors' appointments had run over. I didn't give more detail than that.

THE SURGEON

Dr. ObGyn called to say she wanted me to meet with a surgeon who could remove the calcifications. She wanted to rule out Ductal Carcinoma In Situ (DCIS). Wikipedia informed me that DCIS was a "pre-cancerous or non-invasive lesion of the breast classified as early stage (stage 0). DCIS can be detected on mammograms by examining tiny specks of calcium known as *microcalcifications*. Since suspicious groups of microcalcifications can appear even in the absence of DCIS, a biopsy may be necessary for diagnosis."

I called the surgeon's office and got a message promising a call back. I left a voicemail...but no call back. I called again. Same voicemail. Again, no call back. This went on for more than a week. *Finally,* when the office called me I expressed some of my frustration and the scheduler patiently told me, "I'm sorry—we're just so busy."

Too busy to call someone back who might have cancer? I thought. Apparently, the answer was yes.

I met with the surgeon (Dr. Cutter) and scheduled my surgery date. April 1, 2005—April Fool's Day. This chosen date was my way of maintaining my sense of humor. I knew that until tests were run on the biopsies, there was no way of knowing if I really had breast cancer, but multiple times each day I found myself googling "breast cancer" and reading stuff on the internet I just *knew better* than to read.

THE SURGERY

April 1, 2005 was a Friday. My sister Susan flew in the day before my surgery. First we grabbed dinner with two dear friends at Burma Superstar, a terrific Burmese place in San Francisco. Then we headed to my apartment to meet up with another friend, watch a movie and drink champagne.

I had been given the directive by Dr. Cutter not to drink any liquids after midnight. I drank a beer with my friends at Burma Superstar and when we got home I opened a bottle of Veuve to enjoy with our movie. Then – hell, why not – I opened another bottle just in time to finish drinking prior to midnight. Gah. What is *not* a good idea is drinking too much beer and champagne the night before surgery when Advil and water are off the table after midnight.

With a dull throbbing behind my eyes and a very dry mouth, Susan and I walked to the hospital the next morning to meet with Dr. Cutter, who, similar to my OB-GYN, was a cool, hip gal near my age. I owned up to her immediately that I was hungover and asked if she wouldn't mind directing the anesthesiologist to give me extra fluids in the IV to help me out. She didn't skip a beat and directed the anesthesiologist to fill me up.

Dr. Cutter had me wheeled into the operating room and informed me that she would be putting me into "twilight sleep" rather than under a general anesthetic because the surgery was minor and recovery was easier for the patient. In twilight sleep you're awake but nothing hurts. Everything is easy. In short, *awesome*. The doctors loaded me up on the magical twilight stuff and I was able to talk with Dr. Cutter while she did her work. Mostly what I remember is that I was *very* funny.

After some time, Dr. Cutter indicated to me that she had removed the calcifications and that the surgery was over. I asked her about the lump—and wasn't she going to remove it as well? She said, "No, we're not worried about that—we think it's just a fibrous mass." I told her that *I* was worried about the lump, and it was the reason I had had the mammogram to begin with. I asked if she wouldn't mind simply taking it out. She told me it would be hard for her to identify which part was my lump and which part was regular flesh so in my awesome twilight haze, I volunteered to point it out to her. She agreed to "take a bite" out of it for a biopsy.

DIGGING INTO WORK

I was sore for about a week afterward. At work, I had only told my manager about the surgery so I was super sneaky about my post-surgery recovery. I wore camisoles instead of bras so that the underwire of my bra wouldn't irritate my swollen breast. Over my camisoles I wore button-down shirts each day. This set-up allowed me to slip an ice pack into the camisole. If I wore a baggy enough button-down shirt, I reasoned, no one would notice the ice pack. And no one did. I was so relieved not to need to talk about it with anyone. By the end of the week, I had healed enough to ditch the ice packs.

I really doubled down on work at this point. I was up early every morning for a longer, harder workout and stayed late every night to get my work done. The cancer channel still drummed through my consciousness, but I reasoned that if I had cancer, the pathologists would see it immediately in the biopsied flesh and call me. I kept away from cancer websites and just focused on working and working out.

Cutter called me in mid-April. I was working from home that day and remember slowly sitting down in my armchair to take the call. Dr. Cutter apologized it had taken so long to get back to me with the test results (*two weeks!*). I remember telling her it was okay if she was calling with good news...which she told me she was. "The calcifications and the biopsy of the bite all came back negative."

I didn't have cancer.

And just like that, the cancer channel ceased its transmission.

CHAPTER TWO

WINGWOMAN

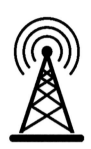

It was December 2006 and there were holiday parties galore. Unfortunately, they all seemed to be scheduled for the same evening. (I don't get how everyone hosts their holiday party on that one Saturday night because they think no one else is hosting a holiday party. Gah.) My girlfriend Katherine and I chose three parties we would attend. We planned to cab between them to let ourselves forget about counting drinks. This is in the land and time before Uber and Lyft, so it was cabs or walking.

The cancer channel was a distant, well-compartmentalized memory. The focus now was on Katherine, who was getting over heartbreak and was quite interested in meeting a man at this party. So when she started a conversation in the kitchen with some guy who had just completed his tenth triathlon (this is San Francisco, after all), I excused myself like any good wingwoman would.

I wandered into a very small room that had just been painted Tiffany blue with chocolate brown accents. I had recently purchased my own condo in the Mission neighborhood of San Francisco, so I was busy assessing whether this particular color scheme would work for my place when the occupants of the room introduced themselves to me. They seemed to be two very lovely married couples. After some polite cocktail-party banter, I resumed my wander through the party.

Predictably, I found myself in front of the cheese. Somehow, I *always* end up in front of the cheese at parties—and frankly, on more than one occasion, I have eaten an inappropriate amount of the hostess's cheese, but once I start, I cannot stop. I love cheese. I mean, I *freaking love cheese.*

So focused on the cheese was I that I hardly noticed when one of the lovely husbands from the very small Tiffany blue room joined me at the cheese table. I suspect I probably tried to stab his hand as he moved in for a piece of brie, but he politely ignored this and told me his name was Geoff and he liked cheese too. We were having that polite, cocktail party get-to-know-you conversation that was surprisingly entertaining when Katherine approached us to tell me it was time to call a cab for the next party.

Geoff said, "You're going to have a tough time finding a cab with the rain. It's also the busiest night of the holiday season and you're out in the boonies...Listen, I had a big night last night and was planning to head home early. I'd be happy to drive you ladies to your next party and just go home from there."

"But what about your wife?" I asked. "Is she ready to leave?"

Geoff looked at me puzzled and said, "I'm not married, and really, I'm ready to leave." Katherine and I quickly decided Geoff would make a great cabbie. I also decided he would be a terrific set-up for Katherine. Once we got into Geoff's car, I, ever the wingwoman, started lobbying him to join us at our party destination.

And he did.

When we got to the party Geoff ran into a friend of his, which allowed me to pull Katherine to the side to share with her my sneaky plan to set her up with this guy, Geoff.

"Totally not my type," she said.

"What? How can this be? He's really cute, very funny, and he must be smart—he went to Stanford! How is cute, funny, and smart not your type!?"

"Not interested," she politely insisted.

I wasn't convinced by her dismissal, so when Geoff joined us later at the party, I lobbied him to drive us/join us at the third party—which he again agreed to. This party was one Katherine had been invited to, and I didn't know anyone there. After about ten minutes at the third party, Katherine decided she was tired of holiday parties and would walk home to her place a block or so away. This whole set-up thing was just not going well. I looked at Geoff and asked if he was interested in staying at a party where we didn't know anyone but one another.

And he was.

We danced, sampled wines on the drinks table, laughed a whole lot, and sometime after midnight, I decided that while I was definitely not going to date a man for at least another year – *maybe* it wouldn't be breaking the rules if I kissed this wonderful man.

And I did.

I was 38 when I met Geoff. By the time we met, I had lived all over the United States—LA, NYC, Boston, San Francisco—moving for jobs I found super interesting and challenging. I had traveled to 35 countries. I had gotten an MBA. I had even gone to culinary school. I was loving my *life adventure*. But what I thought of as my adventure was confusing for some members of my family, like my grandmother. She once told my sister and me that she didn't believe she had ever met sisters who were more different. I knew what she was getting at: my sister Susan had married by 30, settled down in our hometown, had two beautiful daughters, and was taking time off from her teaching career to raise her girls. My sister and her life made sense to my grandmother. Mine did not.

My grandmother had been a nurse who married my grandfather, a neurosurgeon. When she had her first child, my mother Elaine, my grandmother stopped working. Like her parents, Elaine grew up loving science and dreamed of becoming a doctor. As she was finishing her physiology degree from Mount Holyoke and considering applications for medical school, her father told her he had never met a female doctor who was also a good mother.

Reflecting on that, my mother set aside her dreams of becoming a medical doctor and instead got her PhD in physiology. She became a college biology professor who taught her students...and also her children. One such learning related to how pregnancies for women over 35 were high-risk—declining fertility, "old" eggs, health complications like gestational diabetes and hypertension, not to mention the increased risk of miscarriages, birth defects, etc. Given all of those challenges and the fact that I hadn't met my soulmate by 35, I thought perhaps I wasn't meant to have children. I had a great job, a full life, and believed both could continue to be true regardless of whether I got married or had children. I also had a number of terrific friends, both married and unmarried, who didn't plan to have children, so I could envision a life hanging out with them *without children*. I didn't believe my life would be somehow unfulfilled.

And anyway, I had my niece Elizabeth. Elizabeth is my sister Susan's first daughter. She was born in 2001 when I was taking a yearlong sabbatical from my strategy consulting job to go to culinary school and travel. In between those adventures, I spent time at home with Susan and this baby. And I *loved* it/her/everything.

What I learned with Elizabeth is that you don't have to give birth to a baby to love her utterly and completely. I took rolls and rolls of photos of her (because we had film then). I made a photo album of her first year. When she could speak, Elizabeth started calling me "Rah-Rah" because

"Sarah" was too tough. I started calling her "The Monkey" because, well, she was like a little monkey. In fact, I made a mixtape for her first birthday which had all "monkey" songs. The mix had standards like "Five Little Monkeys Jumping on the Bed" and "I Wanna Be Like You" from *The Jungle Book* movie, but also cool songs like Dave Matthews' "Proud Monkey" and Peter Gabriel's "Shock the Monkey." I thought to myself, *Well, if I'm not destined to be a mother, then I am going to be one kickass Rah-Rah.*

Then, when I met Geoff, it seemed like maybe I should rethink my current life strategy.

I remember having sushi with him on one of our very first dates when I brought up the issue of children. We were still in the "hanging out" stage of our relationship where we weren't calling it a relationship, but we were *hanging out* 2-3 times a week. The hanging out stage is a pretty tenuous stage and, in my experience, it is during this stage that things tend to go sideways quickly (perhaps because one party oversteps and brings up children, for example, leading to responses such as "I thought we were just *hanging out*?").

I knew this could be a third-rail topic, but I also felt it was better to get everything out in the open. I suspected Geoff knew my age, but I wanted him to understand the implications of my age if we were going to move beyond *hanging out*. And if my being too old to have children was an issue for him, I'd rather understand that (and break up) three *weeks* into our relationship rather than three *years*. Turns out Geoff's thinking on children was pretty similar to mine. He also questioned whether he would marry (he had just ended a four-year relationship) and wondered if children were in his future. He had nieces and nephews living on the East Coast he would have loved to see more, but he wasn't sure if he would have children of his own.

We then proceeded to date *for two and a half years*. Now don't get me wrong, I think dating for 2 ½ years before getting engaged is just fine when you are in your twenties or thirties—but *as you approach your forties and might want to have children?*

One and a half years into the relationship, Geoff suggested we take a week-long trip to the big island of Hawaii. I was pretty convinced at this point that this was the guy I wanted to marry, so on our first night there, when Geoff suggested I wear the best dress I had packed as he wanted to take me out "for a dinner that would set the tone for the rest of our vacation," I suspected he might be proposing. I kind of went into this out-of-body experience from that moment on as I mentally documented each of the beautiful moments of the night we were getting engaged. We went to the Canoe House in Waimea which is right on the water (mental photo snap). We walked along the beach prior to our reservation (mental photo snap). We ordered mai tais. We ordered our meals. We ate our meals (mental photo snap). And then...we went back to our condo. Geoff had not proposed, and I floated back down to earth.

Two months after the trip to Hawaii, Geoff called me at work to tell me there had been a small fire on the first floor of his apartment building and all residents were being asked to find another place to live for 3-6 months. Geoff asked if he could move in with me for a couple of months...and of course I said yes.

When the management company called Geoff seven months later to tell him it was safe to move back to his apartment, Geoff told me he would probably move back at the start of the month. Surprised, I asked whether he was enjoying living together. He told me, "Yes, of course, but I don't believe that couples who aren't engaged or married should live together."

"Okay!" I said, smiling, "I'm open to that!"

Geoff gave a small smile but told me he wasn't ready to take that step.

As bravely as I could, I asked if his moving out was a signal he was unhappy in our relationship. I asked if it was his gentle way of ending it.

He told me no way, he was happy, he just wasn't ready to commit to marriage.

"Okay," I said, telling myself that I needed to be ready to walk away from this relationship if Geoff wasn't committed to it and I was simply wasting my time.

"Wait. What does 'okay' mean!?" he asked, getting suspicious.

"Okay," I said objectively. "You need to do what works for you and I need to do what works for me."

"Wait. What does *that* mean?" he asked. "I'm not signaling. Don't take this as a signal! I'm fine! We're fine! We're still together!"

"Okay," I repeated. "You need to do what works for you and I need to do what works for me."

"Okay," he said.

Geoff did not move back to his apartment.

A year later, we got engaged and eight months after that – we were married! Given that I was 41 at this point, I immediately made an appointment with a Dr. Fertility at Stanford to see what was possible for us.

AND BABY MAKES THREE?

And so it began. From January 2010 through to January 2012, we tried to get pregnant. I took tests, I had procedures done, I started acupuncture, I injected God-knows-what-drugs into my belly (and a couple of times into my butt). We quickly blew through the $5k in "lifetime" costs my health insurance company allocated to fertility (please note: We were lucky here – *many* couples have no access to fertility insurance what-soever). A friend of a friend gave us her properly-refrigerated leftover fertility drugs. Geoff even sought them out on Craigslist, buying from people who had extra, unexpired supplies they wanted to sell. Pursuing fertility became our primary extracurricular activity. It became a crusade.

After several months of this, I began to notice a pattern. I would inject $1k+ in fertility drugs into my belly to boost my egg production and it would result in...*one* egg. This was the same amount I would have naturally produced without the injections. It was super discouraging and *really* expensive even when we were purchasing the drugs on Craigslist.

In the fall of 2011, I tallied the money we had shelled out in fertility treatments; it was in the tens of thousands. I raised the issue to Geoff and to Dr. Fertility and asked whether it made sense to continue to try to use my eggs. Were we just throwing good money after bad? If Geoff and I wanted to have a baby, I thought we should either find an egg donor or adopt. A *big* decision and not an easy one.

Geoff and I spent weeks talking about the pros and cons of pursuing egg donation. Dr. Fertility referred us to a counselor who specialized in helping couples think through fertility options. If at all possible, I really wanted to carry a baby—to experience a child growing inside me—so my preference was egg donation. I also worried about the long, hard road that would be adoption, so we decided we would explore egg donation first. Should that not pan out, we would look to adopt.

We received a list of agencies who help pair couples with women willing to donate their eggs. We chose the agency closest to us, in Mill Valley, and filled out the paperwork needed for the agency to determine we were sane and suitable for donation. We trekked up to their offices (over a Peet's Coffee) to look at a series of three-ring binders featuring profiles of young women willing to donate their eggs to us. Each woman had submitted a photo and shared her physical traits: brown hair, green eyes, 5' 8", 145 lbs, 23 years old, etc. Each had also filled out a seven-page questionnaire with questions ranging from whether any member of her family has had cancer to what her favorite memory from childhood was and what her life goals were. What was super cool about the questionnaire was that you really could get a feel for the personality of the woman filling it out (assuming she was honest, of course). Geoff and I each grabbed a binder and started reading, pulling out those profiles we thought were the most promising.

I was interested in donors who had brown hair and blue or green eyes so that any child might get Geoff's hazel eyes. I also looked for donors who looked like they could be a relative of mine as I thought that might help our child look like he or she actually fit into our family. And if I'm totally honest, I thought one of the greatest gifts I could give my child is a really good metabolism given that I have always struggled with my weight—so I tended toward women who were "slighter of build" than I. :-)

After a bit, I grabbed Geoff's stack of donors, and as I looked through them I asked him, "Um. Exactly what criteria are you using to select donors?"

"Well...they're cute!" he said with a big grin on his face.

"My love, let me remind you that this isn't a dating decision. You won't be fertilizing their eggs the old-fashioned way. So...why don't we agree on some criteria. It might make this go a little faster," I gently suggested.

We selected donor #805. She met all of the criteria I had laid out (hair, eyes, hopeful metabolism, kinda looked like my cousin). She also loved cooking, listened to music constantly, and liked dogs but not cats (she would fit into our family!). And she spoke three languages. And her father and grandfather were both musicians. This seemed promising— we might have a musical child. We loved the positivity of her application, the fact that the things she liked most about herself were her compassion and her ability to look on the bright side of things. She seemed like someone we would actually like to have as a friend.

Once selected, the agency helped to arrange for donor #805 to meet with Dr. Fertility to go through a battery of tests to ensure her health and viability as a donor. It is a long, expensive process from which there is no guarantee of a baby at the end. Egg donation costs include the agency fee, the donor fee, fertility doctors' fees, fertility drug fees, medical procedure fees, and commuting costs. *Whew*!

We decided not to meet or speak with the donor in order to make it easier on both the donor and ourselves. That said, everyone at the fertility clinic, many of whom we'd gotten to know super well over the 18 months we had been going there, *loved* donor #805. While they absolutely respected everyone's privacy and shared no details about the donor's visits to the clinic, they told us she was upbeat and funny and smart— and they were so excited we were working with her.

The plan then was for donor #805 to take the same fertility drugs I had been taking—see how many viable eggs she produced—and then retrieve those eggs via a very minor surgical procedure that takes between 15-30 minutes. The clinic would then fertilize these eggs with Geoff's sperm, and we would hope some embryos would be created. In parallel, I would be taking drugs to prepare my uterus for implantation of a potential embryo. Once we had fertilized embryos and a fertile uterus, we would schedule an in vitro fertilization, or IVF. We started targeting the end of January 2012. We were so excited! After months of dark disappointment, we could see light.

CHAPTER THREE

WAIT. I HAVE CANCER?

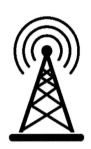

Aside from my fertility campaign, I was also crazy busy with work. I was now running a team called Seller Development that worked with eBay's top 2,500+ sellers to help them better succeed on the platform. Beyond managing a large team, this role meant a lot of travel to trade shows to give talks at industry events and visit with large sellers at their offices, often accompanied by eBay executives.

In both 2010 and 2011, I think I traveled 30 weeks out of 52. It was crazy and demanding beyond anything I had ever experienced before—and I *loved* it. It was one of those jobs where I felt like all of my best skills were being used—my business acumen for sure—but also my ability to relate to and work with all different kinds of people. That said, it was also super stressful because when something went sideways with one of those top sellers (and it often did), I was on the short list of people called to resolve the issue. But I believed so intensely in "enabling economic opportunity for all" that the frantic juggling of my schedule and crazed pace felt like an acceptable trade-off for this noble, higher purpose. I was making a difference in people's lives and that felt important to me.

Then, in September, my HR business partner asked me to interview for a newly-created role at eBay called a "chief of staff" who would be reporting to the newly-appointed president of eBay, Devin Wenig. I wasn't really sure what a chief of staff would be expected to do (or if I even qualified), but I thought to myself, *What can I lose?* I should at least talk with the guy.

Devin is a born-and-bred New Yorker. He is charismatic, intense, and direct—in all of the best ways. From the minute I sat down with him for that first interview, I knew I would love working with him. I interviewed with Devin on a Tuesday. He emailed me on Friday to ask if I could swing by his office. When I sat down in front of him, he said, "I have good news and bad news. The good news is that I'd like to offer you the role as my chief of staff. The bad news is that I need you in London next Wednesday to run a staff meeting."

Um, wow. Okay, then—*game on*.

Clearly my work life was about to change. One of the biggest changes was that I went from being the leader of an extended team of 150+ employees to being an "individual contributor" where I would only be in charge of *me*. Initially, I honestly didn't know what to do with myself. Devin and I were spending our days together talking about eBay, taking trips to various eBay offices (or to visit eBay sellers), and strategizing on what he wanted to accomplish as president. But in those first few weeks, we didn't have a ton of meetings on our schedule, so I thought it would be a great time to get caught up on the routine appointments I had put off during the three years I had been running a big team.

The first appointment I made was with Dr. Dentist for a cleaning. I try to go to the dentist every six months, but since it had been a while, this particular appointment turned into an *hour-long cleaning*. Dr. Dentist and I caught up on what was going on in our lives while she patiently scraped at my teeth.

The week following my teeth cleaning, I noticed a lump on the left floor of my mouth. I had never noticed this lump before and thought one of the cleaning tools Dr. Dentist used must have jabbed me (how did I not notice?). I must have gotten an infection. I called Dr. Dentist to ask if she wouldn't mind taking a look at the lump. She asked me to come in immediately. She felt the lump and suggested a whole spectrum of things it could be from the infection I suspected it was all the way to an extremely rare form of cancer. Dr. Dentist gave me the name of an oral surgeon she wanted me to call in San Francisco. He would take a look at the lump and get me on antibiotics if it was an infection.

I called Dr. OralSurgeon the next day and got on his schedule. When I saw him, he told me he definitely thought it was an infection, and he prescribed antibiotics for the next two weeks. After two weeks, the lump wasn't gone. I called back, but the doctor was on vacation so I would have to wait a month. The lump wasn't painful and didn't seem to be getting any bigger, so it wasn't a big deal at all for me to wait a month. When I saw Dr. OralSurgeon again, he suggested another course of antibiotics and that I get a head and neck MRI (magnetic resonance imaging), just to make sure it "wasn't anything."

It was now December and things at work were starting to heat up. I called the imaging center and was told the earliest appointment was three months out. *Three months*!? Oh my goodness, no way—in three months' time, Devin's schedule would be fully packed and my job would be in full gear. There was no way I wanted to push this off for three months. I simply wouldn't have *time* in three months. The scheduler explained there was a lot of demand at the two MRI locations, so she suggested if I wanted one sooner, maybe I should find another location.

I had already planned a week at home with my family for Christmas, so I found a clinic near my parents' home where I could get an MRI. I remember thinking how efficient I was being by fast-tracking this whole

MRI inconvenience during my vacation. At the clinic, they handed me a CD with my completed MRI. I went immediately to the post office to mail it to Dr. OralSurgeon in San Francisco.

Upon return, I met with Dr. OralSurgeon and cautiously, he told me he didn't like what he had seen on the MRI scan. He told me he wasn't a specialist in this area but he feared what he saw might be a "malignancy." He told me he would refer me to an oral and maxillofacial surgeon who had been a professor of his from dentistry school and *that* guy could tell me what was going on.

I left Dr. OralSurgeon's office and called the maxillofacial surgeon's office on my drive to work. I was told I would have to wait three months *at least* to see him. For the first time, I was uneasy. That word "malignancy" Dr. OralSurgeon had used was banging around in my head. Didn't malignancy mean cancer? Wait. That couldn't mean cancer. I listened to myself telling the scheduler my oral surgeon had referred me because he thought I had a malignancy. Couldn't she please find *some way to get me in to see Dr. Maxillofacial before April*? She said there was a teaching clinic Dr. Maxillofacial was conducting the following week—and she couldn't guarantee I'd be seen—but if I showed up, perhaps the doctor could work me in.

I called Dr. OralSurgeon's office immediately to have them FedEx the MRI CD to the maxillofacial surgeon's office. And with that, I decided to focus on the *really important* health stuff I was working on—namely, the fertility treatments. I did not think about the possibility of cancer again that week. I just wanted to get the whole mystery of what this lump was resolved so I could concentrate on having a baby.

The next week I talked my way into the maxillofacial clinic and found myself sitting in a chair across from the hard-to-schedule Dr. Maxillofacial along with five eager surgeons-to-be hanging on his every word. I remember Dr. Maxillofacial asking me what I did, and when I told him I was chief of staff to the president of eBay, he asked if that was a fancy way of saying I was his secretary. I decided to remain upbeat and friendly with him and get through this exam as quickly as possible. No, he told me, he had not received the MRI CD from Dr. OralSurgeon, but from everything he could feel (or not feel) in my head and neck…this wasn't cancer. He suggested that, just to be safe, I have a biopsy of the lump called a fine-needle aspiration, or FNA. With that additional information he would determine what this lump was and call me on Tuesday of the following week.

I was super relieved to hear from Dr. Maxillofacial that the lump wasn't cancer and happy to do this just-to-be-safe FNA. Geoff and I were going away for the weekend to celebrate his birthday, and it would be terrific to spend that time knowing I didn't have cancer…

Dr. Maxillofacial told me I could walk over to the clinic and have the FNA done immediately. I found the room, showed them the order, and settled down in the pleather La-Z Boy chair. The technician offered me some nasty-tasting, cherry-flavored numbing spray that was meant to anesthetize the area before the test. The taste was worse than any cough medicine I had had as a child, and I really doubted that it was doing any numbing. I was right.

The technician asked me to open my mouth. She leaned in with a syringe that must have had a two-inch needle. I did my very best not to groan out loud as the technician counted to ten as she repeatedly punctured my offending lump. When the technician finally finished counting to ten, she turned away from me to place the sample in the test tubes or whatever. With her back turned, I took a moment to make the face I had been wanting to make during the whole ordeal. I reached up to the side of my face and gently rubbed my jaw, assuring my mouth that now it could begin healing. The worst of it was over. It was then that the technician turned around and said, "Okay, I need to take a second sample now. Are you ready?"

The second time I groaned with every jab.

DIAGNOSIS #1: ADENOID CYSTIC CARCINOMA (ACC)

The week following the FNA, I was preparing for a two-day offsite with Devin's senior leadership team. We would kick off the event with a dinner at a fancy steakhouse and then spend Thursday and Friday hammering through the agenda Devin and I had agreed upon. It was to be my first time in charge of an offsite for the leadership team, and I was eager to do it well.

On Wednesday afternoon, Dr. Maxillofacial called my cell phone but didn't leave a message. I didn't pick up but my phone recognized the number as coming from his medical practice. I quickly ducked into a conference room so as to keep this conversation private and called the number back. Dr Maxillofacial picked up. I think I surprised him with a direct call back but I wanted very much to hear from him what we should do about this not-cancer lump. It wasn't growing quickly, but my tongue would not stay away from it in my mouth, and I was finding it distracting.

Once Dr. Maxillofacial realized it was me, he haltingly told me he had bad news for me. He said something along the lines of, "I'm sorry, Sarah. I know I told you I didn't think your lump was cancer...but it *is* cancer."

Some kind of buzzing started in my head. With as much calm as I could muster, I asked him what kind of cancer it was. As I asked, I began to have an out-of-body experience, but this one was considerably less joyful than the time I thought I was getting engaged. It was more like I was *dis*engaged. My arms felt numb and I watched myself from outside my body as I tried to listen to what Dr. Maxillofacial was saying. What was he saying?

Him: "It's called adenoid cystic carcinoma."

Me: "Can you spell that for me?" (Me trying to use my numb arms to write this out on the whiteboard in the conference room.) "Thank you.

And can you tell me what stage I'm in. I mean...did we catch it early?" The me-person standing outside of me—watching me—was amazed that I was able to keep my voice so calm when, wow, I had cancer. I was amazed that I knew to ask questions like "stage." Did I even know what a stage was? And I knew that it was important to catch cancer early.

Him: "We have no way of knowing what stage you are until we remove the tumor. And do I think we caught it early? I don't know. You've been aware of it since October and it's now January, so it's hard to say if that's early."

Me: "Can you and I remove it tomorrow?" I heard my voice raise a little bit as I began to give into the panic I was now feeling. Wow, *I had cancer.*

The surgeon chuckled softly—f***ing *chuckled*—and told me that he wouldn't be the doctor to perform the surgery, that I needed to be referred to (yet another) specialist who knew more about this cancer than he did.

Me: "Can we call that doctor right now? Can I get on his schedule this week?" I could now hear the panic in my voice. Unbelievable amounts of adrenaline seemed to be running through my body. The buzzing in my head was almost deafening. I wanted to slam down the phone and go running out of the conference room. I didn't know where I wanted to go but I definitely didn't want to be on this call anymore because *wow, I had cancer.* And a really rare, maybe really bad cancer.

The person standing outside of myself told me, "Maintain your dignity, Sarah. Do not let this doctor hear how scared you are." I have no idea why it seemed so important to maintain my dignity when *wow, I had cancer*, but it seemed super important to me at that moment.

Him: "Sarah, I can't control other doctor's schedules. I have no idea when he'll be able to see you or perform the surgery."

Me: "Can you refer me to him?" I was now pleading with this guy.

Him: "Yes. I'll send him a letter with my recommendation of you."

A letter? *A motherf***ing letter?* Okay, so now this scared-self on the phone started to get angry. I had had four months of chasing down multiple doctors and their schedules to try to find out what this lump was, and now that *we know it's cancer* I am being asked to rely on the *postal service* as the referral service to the doctor who may or may not save my life? *No f***ing way...*

That's when Dr. Maxillofacial told me that adenoid cystic carcinoma (ACC) was a particularly rare form of cancer that only 1,200 people in the U.S. are diagnosed with each year, so the doctors didn't know that much about it. I asked what he *did* know about it, especially if he knew anything about survival rates.

Him: "Well, very little work has been done on this cancer because it's so rare, and frankly, there hasn't been a lot of long-term tracking done. We do know that after five years, survivorship is about 80%. After 10 years it drops to around 30%. But this could all be old information. I think there may have been more work done in this field recently, so those statistics may have improved."

A 30% survival rate? Was I going to be dead in five years? Ten years? Was I going to be dead in five months? My panic was rising again. Oh my God, *I have cancer.*

Me: "Dr. Maxillofacial, where can I learn more about this cancer?" My voice was barely above a whisper.

Him: "Well, there's some information on the internet that you can probably read. You're a smart girl, you'll figure it out."

And with that, we hung up.

CHAPTER FOUR

"PROCESSING" MY CANCER DIAGNOSIS

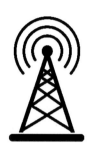

Oh my f***king God, *I have cancer.* No. No no no no.

I could not wrap my head around this. This wasn't supposed to happen. How could I make this *not* true, make it *not* happen? What could I do? I felt helpless and alone. I was terrified. Nothing Dr. Maxillofacial had said to me inspired any sort of confidence that I was going to make it through this. This was a rare cancer. This was a cancer that he, a doctor and an expert, didn't know much about. He didn't know what the *survival rates* were. Were there people who survived this cancer?

My first call after Dr. Maxillofacial was to Geoff. "I have cancer," I told him as matter-of-factly as I could. Unsure what else to do, we agreed to meet at home after my dinner and Geoff's adult league hockey game.

Kristin, the head of human resources for eBay who had approached me about the chief of staff role, stopped by my desk. Kristin is a Tasmanian devil of a human being. She simply operates at a vibration level higher than the rest of us. She is the kind of person who talks through an issue with you—you agree on your next steps—and before you have a chance to put those next steps on your "to-do" list, she has already completed the tasks. Beyond her crazy work schedule, she maintains an active social calendar with multiple dinners per week and yet still manages to remember every birthday and anniversary. And she knows *everyone*—is in regular touch with *all of them* via email/text/phone. She was a force in the universe that I was just beginning to understand. I had told her a week earlier about the lump in my mouth and how I was seeing a specialist to figure out what kind of infection it was.

"Hey, did you ever hear back from that doctor about your lump?" she asked, flashing that upbeat smile of hers.

"Yup," I hedged.

"And?"

"It's not good news." I said, unable to make eye contact with her. I grabbed my iPad and started walking to my next meeting. I couldn't tell her more. I simply didn't know what to say so I walked away.

I was meant to attend a dinner with Devin's executive team that night. I didn't know how to excuse myself from the dinner, what the etiquette might be. "Sorry, something's come up. Turns out I have a rare cancer?" I wasn't sure if I could speak about cancer without losing control in front of these people I worked with and didn't know that well yet. And what if they asked me what was going to happen? How could I answer? I knew nothing about this cancer and what it would do to me. I didn't know what my prognosis was or what my medical treatments would look like. I didn't even have a doctor I was working with. I was just someone who had been told they had cancer and told to figure it out.

After my long drive home, Geoff and I lay side by side in bed. Neither of us slept, but we didn't speak either. We just lay there in bewildered silence.

The next day I drove down to eBay's San Jose office to facilitate an all-day meeting with the executives I'd had dinner with the night before. I had an outline of the agenda and the topics we needed to discuss, but I couldn't concentrate. The drumbeat of "I have cancer, I have cancer, I have cancer" was increasing in volume in my brain and drowning out everything else going on around me.

My cell phone buzzed. I looked down at the number. It was Dr. Fertility calling. I sent it to voicemail. This was the day she was meant to be retrieving the eggs from donor #805.

At the first break, I called Dr. Fertility back and, unbelievably, she picked up. She was excited to tell me how well the retrieval had gone— we had 18 eggs to work with for the IVF we had scheduled for the following week! I told her that was great, but we needed to cancel the IVF because I had salivary gland cancer. She paused and then she softly reminded me how far the salivary gland was from my uterus. She told me we should hold off on implantation of fertilized eggs until after I had received a clean bill of health. She assured me that I was going to make it through this. Boy, did I need to hear that.

Dr. Fertility asked who was going to be treating me for the adenoid cystic carcinoma. I told her how I was being referred to a specialist via the U.S. postal service. She asked if I wanted her to figure out who the top head and neck cancer surgeon was at Stanford. Stanford wouldn't be as convenient, as it was located 37 miles from my home, but I told her that would be *awesome*.

I went back to the meeting and did my best to track what was being discussed. Sometime later my phone buzzed and again it was Dr. Fertility. I excused myself from the meeting to get the name of the top head and neck surgeon at Stanford, a Dr. HeadNeck. Now, in addition to the "I have cancer" earworm in my head, I had questions like when would I be able to call him? Would he take me on as a patient? How quickly would I be able to schedule an appointment? When could we do surgery?

I wanted to crawl out of my skin. I wanted to do *something*. And I realized that as unprofessional as it might be, I needed to leave this meeting and go home and deal with this cancer diagnosis, whatever that meant. I just could not sit in that room any longer.

At the next break, I pulled Kristin into a small conference room and shared my cancer diagnosis news. I told her I was struggling to keep my focus on the day because I was receiving doctors' calls. She listened closely to my disjointed ramblings and asked if I wanted to go home and digest the news. She gently suggested that I should leave if I wanted to, but that I should tell Devin first. She assured me she would cover for me and facilitate the day in my place—that my focus needed to be on doing what I needed to do to get well. Then she hugged me. I cannot begin to express what this kindness meant to me.

I found Devin and asked if we could jump into his office quickly. I saw the concern in his face as we walked into his office and I haltingly told him of my cancer diagnosis. Almost embarrassed, I told him how I was struggling to focus on anything other than that diagnosis. Devin, in his characteristically direct way, simply looked at me and said, "Go home and don't come back until you feel healthy." I apologized for not being able to complete the day, assured him that Kristin would take over for me, and told him I would be in touch as soon as I knew when I could return to work.

He also told me that while he didn't know what all of the rules at eBay were yet, he wanted me to know that I would be taken care of. That there was nothing I needed to worry about from an insurance standpoint. Whatever I needed, he and Kristin would figure it out for me. He, who as a New Yorker was *not* a hugger, hugged me and told me he wished me well.

"Oh, by the way—what kind of cancer do you have?" he said as a total afterthought.

I surprised myself and laughed because I realized we hadn't even discussed that.

I walked back into the conference room where the execs were chatting and waiting for the meeting to start again. I apologized and said I needed to leave, that I had some personal things to take care of. I grabbed my computer and notes and tried to get out of that room as quickly as I could before anyone could ask me anything that would start me crying. "If there's anything I can do to help, Sarah, please let me know," I heard Scott the CFO saying as I ran out of the room.

I swung by my desk to grab my bag and anything else I might want to have at home. I felt like I was evacuating, and I wasn't sure when (or if) I would be back. Cindi, Devin's executive assistant, was sitting at her desk, which was next to mine. I took a deep breath and asked if she had a moment to step into Devin's office. Cindi is this whip-smart, former nursery-school-teacher-turned-executive assistant (turns out the former prepared her remarkably well for working with the latter) who is immensely competent, reliable, trustworthy, empathic, and wickedly funny. If Devin occasionally struggles to show visible emotion, Cindi is his opposite. She is the yin to his yang, which is why they work so effectively together as a team. As I shared my cancer news with her, Cindi's eyes welled up and tears started streaming down her face. My eyes began stinging with the tears I hadn't allowed myself to cry yet. I hugged Cindi and practically ran out of the building.

I cried the entire 57-mile drive back home, at one point pulling over because I was crying so hard my eyes were more closed than open. I called Geoff. I told him I needed him to leave work, for him to meet me at home. He said he'd be right there. Geoff walked into his manager's office to tell her that he needed to leave early—that his wife had just been diagnosed with cancer. She said to him, "Go home and be with your woman. Come back when you are ready." Wow.

At home, Geoff and I sat on the couch. He held me as I sobbed.

As I look back on my reactions in those first few days post-diagnosis, I think I was mostly in shock. And, not having a clear idea of how I *should* be reacting, or really what I could do to control or change the situation, I went into project management mode.

After Dr. Maxillofacial, the surgeon with the, shall we say, less-than-spectacular bedside manner, assured me that I was a "smart girl" and I'd "figure it out," I thought to myself, *Okay, I'm a smart girl. Let me figure this out.* When I arrived home, I started a calling campaign to the head and neck doctor Dr. Maxillofacial had said he would refer me to. The answering service assured me that the doctor was super busy and would look into my case as soon as he had time.

Then I looked up the doctor that Dr. Fertility had said was the top head and neck doctor at Stanford, Dr. HeadNeck. A "Cornelius" on the other end of the line told me that the next available appointment was six weeks from that date—but if an appointment opened up sooner, Dr. HeadNeck would see me.

Six weeks.

The next day, I awoke to messages from both Kristin and Dr. Fertility checking in on me, each letting me know that I was in their thoughts.

Geoff and I got in the car and drove to the medical center's records office to have copies made of all of my medical records. I had discovered that the departments of this particular medical center did *not* share electronic medical files on their patients with one another. Hence Dr Maxillofacial's need to *mail a letter* to the head and neck specialist. *This was 2012*! It was a Friday. I suspect everyone working there just wanted the week to be over, so it took a long time to convince the records office personnel to make physical copies of all of my records. The day was super dreary, rainy and overcast, totally reflecting my mood.

Copies in hand, I walked them to the head and neck specialist's office. I waited in line with the other patients, and when I arrived at the front of the line, I let the receptionist know that I was the Sarah McDonald who had been calling (repeatedly) to make an appointment with the doctor. I told her that I had copies of my medical records to increase the possibility of meeting with the doctor sooner (next couple of days, perhaps?). She smiled patiently and told me the doctor would review my files as soon as he was able. She then placed the records on a discouragingly high pile where I just knew they would get pushed to the side or lost. She then informed me that they would call me to schedule an appointment (i.e. "Don't call us, we'll call you."). As patiently as I could, I said to the receptionist, "I wish I could say to you that this isn't a matter of life or death, but the reality is, *it is*." She smiled patiently again and told me that I should expect a phone call within the next two weeks.

Two weeks. And that was just to schedule the appointment! How much longer would I need to wait until I actually saw the specialist!?

Outside, Geoff was waiting in the car. With the second copy of my medical records in hand, I asked him to drive us down to Stanford. It was absolutely pouring rain as we drove. We hardly spoke. Kristin texted again to check in on me. As we pulled into the Stanford Medical Center parking garage, the rain stopped. We walked cautiously toward the doors of the cancer center and, once inside, we were amazed to hear the sound of a harp wafting its way across the 50-foot-tall (!) lobby atrium. Sunlight was somehow now streaming through the windows and down upon us. Honestly, if angels had been singing, I would not have been surprised. At this moment I knew where I would seek my cancer care. Absolutely

Stanford. We found the concierge desk (*concierge* desk!? Are you kidding me!?) and they directed us across the lobby to Clinic B (past the real-live harpist) where the reception area for Dr. HeadNeck was located.

Again, I waited in line with other patients and when I reached the front, there was this beatific man named Cornelius—the same one who had scheduled me—who greeted me as if we were old friends. I told him that I was hand-delivering my records to Dr. HeadNeck in advance of my meeting with him in six weeks' time. Instead of placing my files behind him in a pile, Cornelius smiled and said, "Well, let me download those records right now!" He popped the CD of my MRI into his computer and magically downloaded it into their database. Then he took the physical copies of my records and placed them in a file that was set on a promisingly small pile for the doctor to review. With that, Cornelius smiled at me and said, "Mrs. McDonald, we will look forward to seeing you in six weeks! In the meantime, I would be remiss if I didn't tell you that we all just gotta give it up to God, you know?"

I was stunned at the kindness of this man. Cornelius looked me straight in the eye—me, the one with cancer—and shared with me what he felt I needed to hear at that moment. He didn't act annoyed by me, he didn't try to rush me along or put me off so he could get to other work or the next person in line. Cornelius paused to connect with me, to respect the pain I was in, to be with me in that moment. For the first time in days, I felt like there was someone who wanted to help me.

I almost kissed Cornelius.

Geoff and I got back in the car and drove home a little less burdened, confident that we were doing as much as we could to move things along. I responded to another text from Dr. Fertility who was checking in on me again and assuring me that she had put in a good word for me with Dr. HeadNeck. At home, Geoff tried to catch up on email while I called my insurance company to inform them that I had just been diagnosed with cancer and that they would likely see more doctor appointments and treatments in my file in the future. It was about 5:30 pm and as the customer service representative, or CSR, was signing me up for a nursing service that would call me weekly to check in on my physical and emotional health, my phone beeped that I had another call coming in. My phone identified this call as coming from "Stanford Medical." I quickly explained to the CSR that I needed to take this call.

"Hi. This is Dr. HeadNeck. I'm a head and neck oncologist at Stanford. Dr. Fertility called me to ask if I would give you a call…so I'm giving you a call."

Oh my God. Here it was 5:30 pm on a Friday evening, and after two days of trying to speak with someone—anyone—who could tell me if I'm going to live or die, this world-famous doctor is calling me directly. I could not believe it. I explained to Dr. HeadNeck that I had just been diagnosed with adenoid cystic carcinoma by another medical center, but was hoping he would be willing to take me on as a patient. He asked me to describe everything I had heard about my diagnosis so far. When I finished, he told me that the cancer sounded small, and that while ACC isn't curable, it sounded like mine was treatable. It would become a matter of "management" for the two of us. Then he told me that he and I would become good friends over many years…

I scribbled notes while Dr. HeadNeck spoke to me. I underlined *good friends over many years*. I told him that I was scheduled to see him in six weeks' time and he told me to call "Maria," and that she would fit me into his schedule for Monday. I thanked him for his time and for fitting me in and I hung up.

I sat down on the floor and could barely catch my breath between body-convulsing sobs. I felt like I had been holding my breath since Wednesday when Dr. Maxillofacial told me I had cancer. For the first time since then I could breathe. I felt as if *no one* would help me

at the original medical center. I was just another patient in a long
line of patients. No one had felt urgency in seeing me or helping me
understand what we needed to do, and now here was this doctor who
was calling me on a Friday night after what was probably a really long
week of seeing other patients like me—and he was making time for me.
He knew how important it was to me to be seen, and he was going to
see me. And my charts. And my scans. Not six weeks from now – but
three days from now. On Monday. He was telling me he would become
my friend over many years.

I texted Dr. Fertility to thank her profusely for calling Dr. HeadNeck.
She suggested that Geoff and I try to distract ourselves over the weekend
by doing something like going to see a funny movie. With no plans
for the evening, Geoff and I checked the listings and saw that *The
Descendants*, a comedy with George Clooney, was playing in the Marina.
Unfortunately, we failed to read the preview prior to jumping in the car
to make the 6:30 showtime.

Okay, so under the heading of "Things not to do when you get a cancer
diagnosis," I would rank in the top three going to see a movie about a
guy whose wife is dying. Granted, there's a lot more to the movie than
just the wife dying (it's a comedy), but it was the worst possible movie for
Geoff and me to go see. At the end of the movie, George has this scene
where he's telling his wife, who is in a coma and on her deathbed, how
much he's loved her. I am quite positive there is more to this scene than
that, but this is all Geoff and I heard. All of the pent-up sorrow I had
been trying to keep under control came hurtling out of me in these loud,
gulping sobs. I looked over at Geoff and he wasn't much better. But you
know the crazy thing? We were so in shock and unable to take care of
ourselves that *we actually stayed until the end of the movie.*

We walked outside and into the too-upbeat nightlife of San Francisco's
Marina district. Geoff pulled me into a doorway and wrapped his
arms around me. After some time, he asked where I wanted to have

dinner and I told him there was no way I could have dinner amidst the lightheartedness of the Marina. I suggested the pizza place in our neighborhood.

We started driving back across the city. As we drove through the Civic Center, near the ballet, opera, and symphony hall, Geoff suddenly pulled over and announced that we were going to see if there was an opening at the bar at Jardiniere.

When you look up Jardiniere in the Michelin guide, it instructs, "For a memorable night on the town, don your best dress, find a hand to hold, and head to this longtime favorite, tinged with a sense of bygone romance. Stop off at the circular bar and join the well-heeled couples sipping cocktails pre- or post-opera." So on this most miserable of Friday evenings, Geoff and I joined the well-heeled at the bar. We distracted ourselves with fancy cocktails and toasted ourselves. We didn't know what the next year would hold, but we told each other that we loved one another and that we would get through it. And for a moment, it felt like things might be okay.

CHAPTER FIVE

ARE YOU KIDDING ME!? WHO GETS TWO CANCERS!?

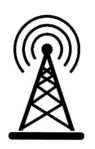

On Monday, Geoff and I drove down to Stanford for my 1 pm meeting with Dr. HeadNeck. We checked in with Cornelius ("So good to see you again, Mrs. McDonald!") and found chairs in the waiting room. As we both booted up our laptops so that Geoff could work and I could pretend to work, we checked out schedule postings to see which doctors were running on time and which were not. Dr. HeadNeck was already 90 minutes behind his schedule, and this was before he fit me in. I felt momentarily guilty for contributing to the schedule chaos but then, with another wave of "I have cancer" panic, I hunkered down for the duration. I would wait all day and night if I needed to.

Two guys sat to my left talking. "Wow, he's really behind today. But you know what? I don't mind. I'm willing to wait as long as it takes to see Dr. HeadNeck." I couldn't help but look over at this guy who was reading my mind. He looked directly back at me and pointed. "Look! She knows what I'm talking about!" I did my best to smile at the man, but as soon as it was polite, I went back to looking at my laptop—which was less intense than looking at a man who might share my diagnosis.

After almost two hours waiting, we were called back to the exam room. Geoff and I reviewed our list of questions and waited. And waited. I sat in what looked like a modified dentist's chair in the middle of the room, and Geoff sat to my side in a tan pleather chair. (What is with all of this pleather in doctors' offices?)

Dr. HeadNeck knocked and entered the room with two others, a nurse and a resident. Dr. HeadNeck was thin and wiry with unruly salt and pepper hair that I suspected was brushed each morning and then ignored for the rest of the day. He introduced himself and his entourage and then leaned back against the wall to begin our discussion. He asked that I remind him of my story—when did I find the lump, how did I come to be diagnosed, what had I heard so far—although he had clearly reviewed everything before walking into the room. Dr. HeadNeck listened so intently that I felt I could almost see his brain working. He had a little twinkle in his eyes as he listened to me, and he joked with Geoff that the greatest challenge we would have post-surgery is whether Geoff would be up to the task of taking on my responsibilities around the house.

He suddenly jumped up and said he wanted to check out the lump. He grabbed gloves and tongue depressors and asked me to open my mouth. After he had prodded my lump with his finger and felt around the floor of my mouth, he repeated everything he had said to me on the phone. He told me this was one of the smallest tumors he'd seen in his 20+ years and that while the cancer was incurable, it was treatable. We would remove the tumor and then we likely wouldn't even need radiation. I asked if we could remove the tumor that week, and Dr. HeadNeck gently told me he had other surgeries scheduled and that I needed to stop taking pills like aspirin, fish oil, and my beloved Advil for at least two weeks before the surgery because they would impair my body's ability to clot blood. He assured me I would be scheduled as soon as possible, however. I asked our litany of questions and Geoff furiously typed the answers into our iPad.

I had walked into that appointment so frightened that Dr. HeadNeck was going to confirm the death sentence I knew I had been given. I had whispered to my frightened self all of the assurances Dr. HeadNeck had given me over the phone on Friday night, but I was convinced none of it would hold true once he had seen my scans. But that's not what he said. Without giving me guarantees, he told me he thought it would be okay. He told me we would know one another for a long time. I felt my body relaxing and easing back into the world of the living. I felt the warmth of the sun again. I saw the wind blowing through the grasses as we walked back to the car. We called all of our family members on the drive home to tell them this great news.

SURGERY #1

As promised, my surgery was scheduled two weeks after my initial appointment with Dr. HeadNeck. On the day of the surgery, Geoff and I were asked to show up at 6 am (!) for a 10 am surgery appointment. *What!?* We live a freaking *hour away* from the hospital. 4:30 am was bleak. I was so bleary eyed I was lucky I was wearing pants when we arrived at the hospital. We had been told not to bring any valuables, but that I would need to show my ID. I thought this was pretty funny because who in their right mind is going to impersonate me and *willingly* have a doctor remove their salivary gland? But I guess the hospital wants to make sure they have the right person. And you know what? I totally forgot to bring my ID and didn't realize it until we were parking in the lot and Geoff said, "You have your ID, right?" Gah.

We momentarily discussed driving home to get the ID. I decided that was crazy and that I would just talk them into operating on me. Lucky for me, they agreed.

I suited up in a hospital gown and was given an IV. We signed papers and quickly met with Dr. HeadNeck, who seemed excited for his day of surgeries as evidenced by the twinkle in his eye on high beam. I was wheeled into a surgery room, scooted from my gurney onto a surgery bed, and asked to count back from ten as the anesthetic in my IV gently put me to sleep. When I woke up, I could not beg for water fast enough. The back of my throat was parched beyond what I thought was possible. The nurse kindly gave me a cup of ice chips to help relieve the pain.

Dr. HeadNeck swung by and told Geoff and me that the surgery had gone well and he believed he had achieved "clean margins." This meant he believed he had removed *all* of the cancer cells in my mouth. Geoff and I thanked him and thanked him again as I was wheeled upstairs to my shared hospital room. The woman I was to be sharing the room with was already in her bed and had undergone some kind of esophageal surgery earlier in the day. She was alone, and she was suffering. We wanted to give her privacy but wow, was it difficult to listen to the labored gurgling from her side of the curtain. And if I'm honest, it completely freaked me out. I did not wish to be callous to this other human being and her suffering, but I could not stay in that room for the night. I started lobbying the nurse to allow me to go home, and after I proved I could walk up and down the hall on my own and use the restroom, she did.

DIAGNOSIS #2: INVASIVE DUCTAL CARCINOMA

I met with Dr. HeadNeck two weeks after the surgery so he could see how the wound was healing. He poked and prodded in my mouth and asked how Geoff's increased home responsibilities were coming along. Then he shared with us that while he had believed he had achieved clean margins at the time of surgery, the radiologist reviewing the scans worried that some cells might be making their way to my nerve (referred to as "perineural invasion"). The best way to ensure all cancer cells were killed would be to radiate the area over a six-week period.

Dr. HeadNeck told me the side effects of radiation to the mouth were not insignificant and could include moderate-to-severe mouth sores, dry mouth, etc., so we should consider whether I wanted to radiate or not. (I had a choice!?) Geoff and I assured Dr. HeadNeck that we wanted to be as aggressive with this cancer as possible, so I was ready to go through whatever I needed to go through physically if it meant killing the cancer once and for all.

"It could mean dry mouth," Dr. HeadNeck said, looking at me very directly.

"Dry mouth for six weeks?" I said confidently but with no reason whatsoever for that confidence. "I can handle that."

"No. Dry mouth for the rest of your life," he said quietly and then paused to let that sink in.

I thought about my parched throat on the day of the surgery and wondered if that was going to be a regular occurrence if we radiated. Grimly, I said, "I want to be as aggressive as we can be. If it results in dry mouth, I'll figure it out."

I had a whole new list of questions on my iPad ready for Dr. HeadNeck that day. Over the past couple of weeks, I had been reading about cancer and wanted to understand as much as I could about ACC and what I could be doing to ensure it didn't recur. Were there certain foods I should or shouldn't eat? (Answer: Just eat *real food*.) Could I do periodic blood tests that would show markers to tell us that the cancer had returned? (Answer: No.) How often should I do MRIs to scan for progression of the disease? (Answer: Annually, possibly less often the farther we get from initial diagnosis.)

My final question was one I hesitated to ask because I feared it made me sound like a hypochondriac/paranoid person now that I had had a cancer diagnosis. I asked him whether the lump in my left breast that had been biopsied in 2004 should get checked out again. If the salivary gland cancer was so slow growing, could it be that the lump in my breast was actually a metastasis of the salivary gland cancer? Had my cancer, in fact, spread?

Dr. HeadNeck shook his head. "Not likely. When ACC travels, it likes to spread to the brain or the lungs (me: oh God), not to the breast. So if the lump in your breast was cancer, it would likely be breast cancer. But Sarah, you already have one of the rarest cancers out there. The likelihood that you have two totally unrelated cancers at the same time? We just don't really see it in someone so young. But if it will make you feel better, you should get it checked out with your OB-GYN."

Dr. HeadNeck's response—which I'm sure was based upon his 20+ years of working on head and neck cancers—felt discouraging. He didn't call me a hypochondriac, but I did get the impression he thought I was overreacting. And to be clear, I had been told by top physicians at the other medical center that I did *not* have breast cancer, so it was very reasonable to think I was overreacting. But I thought to myself, I have a week before I go back to work—why don't I just get the lump checked out by my OB-GYN. It couldn't hurt, and it would put my breast cancer fears to rest.

Since the cancer scare in 2004, I had had an annual mammogram each year, and each mammogram had come up "clean." Beyond regular self-exams, I also met with Dr. ObGyn annually and had a breast exam and pap smear. Fighting against my embarrassment and fear that I was being a hypochondriac, I called Dr. ObGyn's office. I shared that I had recently been diagnosed with salivary gland cancer and that I would like to meet with the doctor to discuss a worrying lump on my left breast. The receptionist told me that Dr. ObGyn's next available appointment was in six weeks. *Six weeks.*

I took the appointment and then immediately started searching for Dr. ObGyn's email address in my contacts. Thankfully, I had it. I emailed

Dr. ObGyn directly to tell her about that ACC diagnosis and to ask that we revisit my breast lump. Her team had told me I needed to wait six weeks—was there a way to see her sooner? She emailed back to suggest we meet the following Wednesday at 8 am before her schedule began (and, incidentally, before she was going for her own mammogram). It was also the first day I was scheduled to be back at work, so I emailed Devin to let him know I'd be a little tardy that day.

When I met with Dr. ObGyn she felt the lump and asked, "Has this grown?"

"No."

"I looked at your charts this morning. All of your mammograms have been clean. Hmm. You have very dense breast tissue—we should probably do an MRI because sometimes mammograms don't show tumors on women with dense breast tissue."

What!? How is it that we had never discussed having an MRI? I tried my best to listen to *everything* Dr. ObGyn was telling me, but I had a sinking feeling in my stomach. I reminded Dr. ObGyn that Dr. Cutter had "taken a bite" out of the lump in my left breast to do a biopsy and it had come up clean. I pointed to the scar on my breast. Dr. ObGyn took a look at the scar and then pointed out to me how far the surgery scar was from the lump we were discussing. She looked directly at me and said, "I'm not sure the surgeon got a bite out of the lump."

Suddenly, I had electricity running through my whole body. I looked down at the scar and the lump and *for the first time* noticed how far they were from one another. I really cannot explain or understand how it is that neither Dr. ObGyn nor I had ever noticed this before. Maybe I just wanted to believe that the lump wasn't cancer so it was easier to just dismiss it as the fibrous mass the doctors had told me it was? But now we were both looking down at my breast and realizing the lump may never have actually been biopsied. Maybe they had made a mistake and biopsied healthy flesh. Maybe they'd missed it eight years ago. Maybe I had breast cancer too. Oh my f***ing God.

"I will order you an MRI," she promised me. I relayed to her my experience of being told the first available MRI appointment was three months out. She told me that as a doctor, she'd be able to get me one sooner at her medical center. When she called back later in the day, she had been given an appointment for me six weeks out. There was *no way* I was going to be able to handle waiting six weeks to find out whether I had breast cancer too. Instead, I called Stanford Hospital and was given an appointment for the following Monday.

Now back at work, I kept replaying my conversation with Dr. HeadNeck where he told me how unlikely it was that I had two primary cancers. I also tried not to think about how many years I had had that breast lump. How long does cancer take to spread to other parts of the body? I didn't know, but eight years of potential cancer in my breast didn't seem like it would be a good thing.

After only being back at work for three days, I left work early to go for the breast MRI. The big difference in this MRI experience was now, instead of being face up when I was conveyor-ed into a small tube, I was asked to lie face down with my breasts hanging freestyle in the hole cutouts they had fashioned in the conveyor bed. Totally weird.

Once the 45-minute MRI was completed, I sat in a waiting room, slightly dazed from the banging of the MRI and still in my hospital gown, while Dr. Radiologist reviewed the pictures. I was then called into a private room to speak with Dr. Radiologist, who explained to me that she'd like to get a sonogram, and possibly a biopsy, of the lump. Again I was ushered back to the waiting room to stare at inspirational posters until another technician took me into yet another exam room.

This technician asked me to lie on my side on a padded exam table while she moved a lubricated sonogram wand over my lump and looked at the pictures on her monitor.

"Wow, that's really big, huh?" she said to me with what I heard as both shock and concern. I quietly nodded at her.

She then put the wand into my armpit and took photos there.

Dr. Radiologist joined us and the technician shared the photos of what I learned was a 4.5 cm lump. The technician and radiologist then discussed what I heard as "lymphatic involvement" and the technician showed the radiologist the photos she had taken from my armpit of two swollen lymph nodes. The radiologist told me they'd like to take a "core biopsy" of the lump. The core biopsy was different from the fine needle aspiration (FNA) procedure for the tumor in my mouth. With an FNA, they use a needle to extract the cells. With a core biopsy they wanted to extract more than just cells in order to run tests. A bigger sample means a bigger instrument—and much, much more noise. They injected me with some anesthetic and then used an instrument that looked like a staple gun to me to (thwap! thwap! thwap!) extract flesh from my lump.

As we finished the tests, tears started running down my face as I knew in my heart that I had breast cancer too. And while I may have caught the ACC in my mouth early, there was *no way* I had caught the breast cancer early. This lump had been around since 2004, and it was now 2012. Eight years. Eight years I had been walking around with breast cancer that the doctors and I had missed.

When the technician saw that I was crying, she asked if they were hurting me or if the biopsy was painful. "No," I said as bravely as I could.

I drove home in a trance.

When I arrived home Dr. ObGyn called me. She told me Dr. Radiologist had called to say she didn't like what she saw in my scans. We would still need to wait a couple of days for the results of the biopsy to come back, but Dr. ObGyn wanted me to know sooner than later that it was likely breast cancer.

"Why is this happening?" I asked, feeling defeated and helpless.

"I don't know," she said.

I hung up with Dr. ObGyn and immediately called Kristin.

"I am still waiting to get the tests back, and I won't hear until next week, but it looks like I have breast cancer too, Kristin. I think I'll need to go back out on leave and I don't know when I'm going to be coming back to work."

She told me how sorry she was to hear that, and I could hear in her voice that she really meant this. She assured me the last thing I should worry about right now is work—that I should just focus on getting the treatment I needed. She told me that she'd have the benefits team call me the following week to handle the paperwork that would extend my leave. She told me she would be thinking of me and that I should call if I need anything. "I mean that, Sarah" she said.

I tried not to think about what it would mean to have two cancers. Was this just the beginning of what would be a whole bunch of cancers? How long do people live with two (or more) cancers? The "I have cancer" drumbeat was deafening in my head. I felt like I was in fight or flight mode every hour of every day. I started to wonder if it is possible to have a heart attack from stress. While I felt prepared for whatever physical pain I might experience with radiation, etc., I wasn't sure I was going to be able to sustain the level of stress I was feeling. For the first time in my life, I started thinking I needed to be medicated to calm down. I vowed to ask the next doctor I met with to prescribe something to give me some relief, a break from my terror.

On Thursday, I had a preliminary appointment scheduled to meet with Dr. RadOnc (this is an abbreviated version of her full job title which is "radiation oncologist" but clearly this nickname wins the contest for best abbreviated-to-protect-her-identity doctor name). As Stanford is a teaching hospital, I first met with one of her residents to review my charts before Dr. RadOnc would meet with me. The resident, a young man in his mid 20s, started reading from my chart on the computer. He ran through my prior medical history and detailed the treatment of my adenoid cystic carcinoma. Then he said, "Oh, and I see you've had a positive diagnosis for breast cancer as well?"

"Um, well, I guess I have now," I said to him.

"What?" he said with this panicked look on his face. "You haven't been told you have breast cancer?"

"Nope, but I appreciate you confirming what we already suspected."

I am sure it was a total bummer for him as a new resident to discover that he'd just given someone a cancer diagnosis by accident, but somehow, it seemed funny to Geoff and me in a gallows humor kind of way. I told the resident not to worry about it. It wasn't his fault I had two cancers.

Dr. RadOnc joined us and explained that there would be a slight delay in starting my radiation therapy on my mouth now that there was a confirmed second cancer. The doctors who would treat each cancer would want to discuss how they could coordinate that treatment.

That afternoon I received a phone call that I had an appointment scheduled with a Dr. BreastOnc (breast oncologist) and a Dr. PlasticSurgeon (breast plastic surgeon) for the following week. I was beginning to lose count of the number of doctors I was meeting and working with at Stanford alone. 7? 8?

Dr. BreastOnc's office was in the building across the street from the building with the 50-foot-high ceilings and the harps where Dr. HeadNeck's office was located. We were taken into a small room that had a padded examining table. I jumped up on the table and Geoff sat on a chair to the side. We were introduced to Dr. BreastOnc, Dr. PlasticSurgeon, at least two residents, and one nurse. With seven people crammed into an exam room normally meant to have only one doctor and one patient, we practically needed air traffic control any time one of us moved a limb. After shaking hands with each of them, Dr. BreastOnc stood in front of me and touched my legs that were dangling over the exam table. I was so jumpy and nervous with anticipation of what they were going to tell me that I retracted from her touch. I was surprised by my strong emotional response to her touching me and hoped she hadn't noticed.

Dr. BreastOnc looked directly at me and started, "I understand you've already heard that the biopsy you received last week indicates that you have breast cancer. The good news, if there is good news with a breast cancer diagnosis, is that you have estrogen-positive, progesterone-positive, HER2 negative breast cancer. This is the most common form of breast cancer and one we know how to fight. We know the treatments that work for this breast cancer, and we believe we can speak in terms of curing you of this cancer."

My God, this was not what I was expecting to hear. I had thought I would be told there was little they could do now that there were two cancers. Instead, they told me there was very good reason for me to have hope.

What a wholly different experience receiving this breast cancer diagnosis versus the ACC diagnosis, both in terms of delivery as well as prognosis. With my ACC diagnosis, Dr. Maxillofacial had called me on the phone to tell me I had a cancer so rare and incurable that he wasn't familiar enough with it to give me reliable information, and that I would need to figure it out myself. With my breast cancer diagnosis, I had a packed room of doctors gathered around me, touching my leg while they spoke with me, telling me they had a plan for my treatment and they believed they would cure me.

Dr. BreastOnc was eager to use a relatively new protocol that would have me doing chemotherapy first (neoadjuvant chemotherapy, to be exact) to break down my tumor and "erase the footsteps of cancer" that might have trekked throughout my body, then surgery to remove the tumor. She also liked this protocol as I would be able to receive treatments for both cancers concurrently (radiation for ACC and chemo for the breast).

Dr. PlasticSurgeon walked through the pros and cons of lumpectomy versus mastectomy (single, double). (Note that Dr. PlasticSurgeon would be doing the surgery regardless of whether it was a lumpectomy or a mastectomy because he's the guy who has the skills to "preserve the breast".) I told him I was absolutely positive that I wanted a double mastectomy because I wanted the breast cancer gone completely from my body. He spoke to me of survival rates for both decisions and suggested that since we were doing chemo first, I would have some time to weigh the options. "A mastectomy is major surgery," he told me. "And once the surgery is complete, you can't change your mind or reverse your decision. Lumpectomy is an option in your case, and not everyone has that option. Mastectomy is something we could hold for a future option if we need it."

Future option? *No f***ing way*, I thought. I am doing this once and we are getting rid of these cancers and then I am going back to my normal life.

The doctors told me they'd be conferring with doctors HeadNeck and RadOnc and would call me back in with a coordinated plan once everyone was aligned. Meanwhile, they asked that I schedule a CT scan and a bone scan to see if the breast cancer had spread. They also said they'd be contacting the genetics team to meet with me as they don't often see two primary cancers like this and they wanted to understand if this was part of a "larger story."

We walked out of that room so full of hope. The ACC was small—incurable but treatable. The breast cancer was common and curable. We could treat them at the same time. How could we possibly be so lucky? We now understood that I would have months of treatments, and that some days would probably be hard, but there would be another side to this mountain. And on the other side—well, maybe there could be a baby.

IT'S JUST TOO MUCH

Dr. BreastOnc called me three days later to ask if Geoff and I were available to meet with her. She said she had some things she wanted to discuss with us prior to beginning treatments.

We met Dr. BreastOnc in the same room we had met with the team of doctors to discuss my diagnosis and potential treatment plan. I was perched on the examining table again and Geoff was to my right in one of the two metal chairs in the room. Just as she had the first day, Dr. BreastOnc walked into the room, walked up to me, and immediately started rubbing my legs.

In order to rub my legs, Dr. BreastOnc stood in my personal space – but it wasn't off-putting. She radiated kindness. She had shoulder length light brown hair that was tied back into a low ponytail. Her voice was soft but firm with a slight accent revealing her New Jersey roots. Her blue eyes looked at me so intensely that I felt she was seeing into my most private thoughts – like she might have an inkling of how much I had been suffering.

"You've both had a lot to process over the last couple of weeks. How are you doing?" she asked gently.

Given the "treatable" and "curable" news from our last couple of appointments, Geoff and I were feeling reasonably upbeat and optimistic and we said as much to Dr. BreastOnc.

"Listen, I read in your charts that you were pursuing fertility treatments at Stanford when you were first diagnosed with the ACC. Is that right?"

"Yes," I told her. We'd been meeting with Dr. Fertility for the last two years, had made the tough decision to find an egg donor, and were planning on an IVF cycle at the end of January. I told her we had canceled that due to the ACC diagnosis, but that we now had 16 viable embryos sitting on ice.

"What have you heard about your fertility options at this point?" she asked.

I told her that our fertility doctor was the first person I spoke to about my ACC cancer diagnosis after Geoff. Dr. Fertility had thought that perhaps in two years, after my cancer treatments were finished, we could schedule an IVF and try again to get pregnant.

Dr. BreastOnc looked me directly in the eyes and shook her head at me.

"I believe your breast cancer diagnosis will impact that plan. Once your breast cancer treatment is completed, I will prescribe a drug for you called tamoxifen that blocks estrogen, which is critical in pregnancies. I will want you to take that drug for the next ten years to prevent a recurrence of your breast cancer, which means we wouldn't want you to be pregnant for the next ten years. Ten years from now you'll be 55, and I don't believe you will be eligible for IVF treatments. You won't be able to carry a baby."

I just kept looking at Dr. BreastOnc and blinking as I processed what she was saying. "Oh," I said and immediately began berating myself silently for having gotten my hopes up. I had two cancer diagnoses. I should feel lucky that they were treatable and that I could reasonably hope to be alive by the end of the year. Who was I to wish for a child?

I looked at Geoff sitting next to me and could see tears welling up in his eyes. "It's just too much," he said softly, his voice shaky with emotion.

Dr. BreastOnc apologized for having to be the one to deliver this tough news. She spoke about there being many different ways to create a family, and that perhaps after we had had time to process all of this information, we could consider those other options. Then she offered to leave the room and give us some privacy.

That day it felt like cancer had killed all of our dreams.

CHAPTER SIX

THE CANCER BOMBSHELL

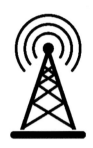

The words "I have cancer" were a verbal hand grenade the first couple of times I said them out loud. On my worst days, I would reprocess my diagnoses in front of the person I was speaking with, which made for ugly contortions as I fought the tears on the battleground of my face. Equally ugly, awkward, and unpredictable could be the reaction of the other person to my news—followed by *my reaction* to *their reaction*. One close friend from business school began sobbing uncontrollably in her elegant NYC executive office when I spoke with her (my reaction to her reaction: I cried harder), while another friend awkwardly asked me if I was "learning anything" from the experience (my reaction: I tried not to slug said friend). It was all very unpredictable and out of control, and I had no idea how to do it differently.

There was also a big part of me that was somehow *embarrassed* that I had cancer. Saying I had cancer seemed like an unseemly admission of mortality. Like the wounded animal in the pack, I didn't want folks to leave me behind now that I had a potentially fatal flaw—conclusive impermanence. What I really wanted was to power through my treatments, get past this small cancer hiccup, and possibly forget this had ever happened. I wanted my (normal) life back. That was my goal.

Geoff and I thought we should tell our families as soon as we could so they could know what we were going through, support where they could, and be part of our "team." Neither one of us lived near our parents, so this meant the news needed to be shared over the phone. My initial cancer diagnosis was on a Wednesday and we called our families on Sunday.

What I didn't anticipate was this:

Geoff and I had been going through fertility treatments for almost eighteen months by the time of my first cancer diagnosis. We had been through multiple cycles at that point, and rather than subject our parents to the rollercoaster experience of the fertility journey, we had stopped giving them any updates. We didn't tell them when we were in a "cycle" so they wouldn't be disappointed when it didn't work (again). So when we called my parents to tell them we had some health news, the first words out of my mother's mouth were, "Oh, this is the call we have been praying for!" Ugh.

Once I awkwardly shared our devastating news, my parents wanted to know what the prognosis was and what treatments I would be undergoing. All reasonable questions to which, on the Sunday after my diagnosis, we had no answers. We hadn't even met the doctor yet, much less spoken about treatments available to me—and we certainly had no idea how aggressive my cancer was or would be. Promising to call as soon as we had more answers, we then defeatedly hung up the phone. And then, because we were in shock and not thinking clearly, we proceeded to make it worse by calling Geoff's parents. His mother, whose sister had died two years earlier of brain cancer, excused herself when she started crying. Geoff's father was at a loss as to what to say so the phone call ended as awkwardly as it had started.

This was not going well.

I wish I could tell you that we got smart after that and didn't call anyone else. Nope. We proceeded to call both of Geoff's brothers and then my brother and sister. The calls were quick, tough on everyone, and short on answers. Our news was so surprising to everyone that I don't think anyone knew what to ask, and when they asked, we didn't have any answers. It was a communications trainwreck. Our lack of answers on Sunday also meant that once we saw Dr. HeadNeck on Monday, we had to call each of those families back to tell them the latest and try to field any and all questions that had come to them in the past 24 hours. It was awful.

After the horror of sharing the news with our families over the phone, we decided anyone else we would tell would be in person. Geoff and I made the decision that we would keep the circle small— limit it to family, friends we saw most frequently, and the people we worked for. That's it.

Strangely enough, I remember very few of those first conversations now in part because I think I was in such a haze of adrenaline. I only remember bits and pieces, like when you're trying to eavesdrop on a conversation in the other room and you only pick up every other word. Sometimes you can figure it out, and sometimes you're just left with word salad.

Totally ignoring my commitment to tell close friends in person, I called my friend Tripti. Tripti and I met when we were 24 and worked for the same company. I was living in NYC and she lived in Houston, and we met when email was just becoming a thing. Then she moved close to where I lived and then away again—and then I moved close to where she lived and stayed. She went to culinary school. I went to business school. She joined a startup and left when she realized it was crushing her soul. I left consulting for similar crushed-soul realizations and joined a tech company. Tripti now did yoga full time and I did Powerpoint.

The only thing I remember from telling Tripti I had cancer is that she said to me, "I am so glad to hear you'll be getting treatment at Stanford for this cancer. Let's call them *Team One*—they're your Western medicine team. I'd like to be in charge of *Team Two*—your Eastern medicine team. Will you let me do that?"

Yes. Yes, of course.

I set up time with Tripti for the following week to begin my Eastern medicine regime. She wanted to give me a one-on-one yoga session to get us started, and she wanted to explain a number of other therapies she thought would be helpful for my healing from cancer treatments including yoga, loving-kindness meditation, and acupuncture.

ONE-ON-ONE YOGA PRACTICE

My friend Tripti has a special room in her home for her yoga practice. It is a serene room where once you close the door, all sounds from her home disappear. You cannot hear her Bernese Mountain Dog, Otis, bounding up and down the stairs or playing with his stuffed toys. You cannot hear her husband, Todd, tapping away at the computer or running a conference call or trying to find the words to tell my husband who has come with me how sorry he is that I have cancer and ask how he can help.

The first thing you notice when you walk into Tripti's practice room is the small shrine she keeps with a statue of the Hindu deity Ganesh. Tripti will tell me that "Ganesh is known to place obstacles in front of us so that we may overcome them, and learn and grow as people." But I don't know this yet. There is also a bookcase filled with books on yoga and meditation. And there are mats and pillows and foam blocks stacked against the wall to support anyone in this serene room who wishes to practice their yoga.

Given that my prior yoga practice was limited, Tripti began this first session gently. We focus first on breathing. We breathe in and we breathe out. We breathe over five counts. We breathe for a long time. I try to match my breathing to hers. And I try to focus on her voice only. Not the voice in my head that is chanting the "I have cancer, I have cancer, I have cancer" mantra, but instead this soothing voice of my friend who is willing me to breathe.

She shows me how to do "child's pose." Down on all fours—now put your feet together and allow your knees to push out and create a triangle with your legs. Now lower your butt to your feet and bring your hands together and extend your arms forward. Allow your forehead to touch the ground. Sink into the pose. Breathe. Breathe. Good. Hold the pose. Breathe through the pose. Breathe. Good.

What Tripti doesn't know is that I had been doing this pose all week without knowing it was child's pose. It is the pose my body has intuitively taken—a kind of modified fetal position—as the waves of sobs passed through me and I mentally tried to get my head around the fact that I have incurable cancer. Incurable. Cancer.

From child's pose, Tripti has me transition into a seated position with my legs in front of me, now forming a gentle square as the bottoms of my feet touch and my knees become the sharp opposing points of the square. At first I am just able to keep that position with my hands draped lightly on my sharp knees. I breathe, we breathe. Seconds and minutes go by. Tripti tells me to be concerned only with what is right here in front of me. What is right now. I try to focus on getting this one thing right.

We deepen this pose by bending over our bodies, our legs, our gentle squares with sharp knees. I am a pretzel of limbs. I am a clam that is closed tight. I am a child hiding a secret. I am a woman terrified that she has cancer who is just trying to breathe through the appointments, breathe through the tests, breathe through the treatments, breathe through this pose.

I note that my heart has slowed and I have lost track of time. I have lost so much this week: my health, my perceived immortality, my innocence, my dignity. When my world came to a screeching halt with my diagnosis, somehow, inconceivably, it continued for everyone else. Everyone else is going about their lives and naively believing they have time enough to waste while I wonder if I will still be breathing in and out a year from now.

We end this first yoga practice together sitting with our legs crossed and our hands pressed together in prayer close to our hearts. Tripti says some beautiful words about time taken in practice being a gift to one's self and about being a light in the world, and then ends with "namaste." In Hindi, this word means "I bow to the divine in you." I've always suspected many people who say "namaste" do so without truly understanding what it means. Tripti means the phrase sincerely and we bow to the divine in one another. Once we have finished our practice she looks directly in my eyes and asks how I am doing. At the surface she is asking how the yoga practice was for me, but I know what she is really asking is what is going on in my head and in my heart.

Even when you have spent countless evenings/weekends/years sharing your lives across decades, somehow there are subjects that are still taboo between close friends. Dying and Death are two of them.

"This is a safe space, Sarah. You can say whatever you need to say."

"I know," I said. I could feel all the things I needed to say lining up in my throat—pushing and shoving one another to be the first one out of my mouth. I wanted to shove them back down. I wanted to gulp them into my stomach where it was too far for them to climb back up and out and be seen for the ugly, small thoughts they were. I wanted to tamp them down so they couldn't trigger the tidal wave of emotions threatening to breach my levee of control. I feared once they were said, my thoughts, my fears, my new reality couldn't be unsaid. It/they/this would be true.

Of course we all die. *Of course*, we *all* die. I just didn't want it to be true for me. Not now. Maybe not ever.

I lose my battle with my ugly, small thoughts and they come pouring out of me in no coherent order. I lay them in front of her like I am laying out photos of myself naked. I am ashamed and yet once I start, I cannot stop. I am saying aloud all of the thoughts that have left me prone in my bedroom for the last week. I find myself climbing into that prone position as I whisper my darkest fears to her.

"I don't know how to do this. I don't know how to say or do *any* of this. I don't know how to die at 44. I don't know if this is the last year of my life and if it is, what does this year look like? I know I have a high threshold for pain, but I don't know how much dying is going to hurt. Can I handle it? Beyond the physical pain, I'm not sure I can handle the emotional pain. Right now I'm so stressed out that I'm not convinced I won't die of a heart attack before the cancer can have a chance to kill me. I'm honestly losing my mind. I can't eat. I can't sleep. And all I keep thinking is: I have cancer. If I have to die now—this year—is there a way that I can die gracefully, not embarrass myself? If I have to die, I desperately want to die well, without hysteria and loss of dignity. And I just don't know if I can do that because I'm just so scared. I'm so scared."

My voice was shaking. My whole body was shaking. I don't know that I have ever been more vulnerable with another human being.

I don't think Tripti tried to tell me that everything was going to be okay, or that it would be different from what I was describing. She listened and she cried with me. And she promised to be with me regardless of the outcome. She promised that we would take everything one step at a time. She would be the captain of *Team Two*. She would help me breathe.

TELLING FRIENDS

Geoff and I began meeting friends for dinner, brunch, or coffee to share the "I have cancer" bombshell with them. I even worked up a little script for myself to help keep me focused as I told them about the cancer:

I have some really tough personal news I need to share with you. I've been diagnosed with a really rare form of cancer called adenoid cystic carcinoma, or more simply, salivary gland cancer. We, including the doctors, don't know a lot about it because only about 1,200 people are diagnosed with it each year. We're still in the early stage of understanding what the treatments will be for me, but likely it will include surgery and radiation. And yes—we're totally freaked out about it but wanted to tell you as soon as we could. I would be happy to answer any questions you have, if I know the answers.

The first person we met with for dinner was one of my best friends from business school, Alex. He loves food like we love food, and so he had suggested a new trendy neighborhood restaurant with dark booths (terrific) and small portions (less terrific). Geoff and I dressed in hip, cool city clothes and I stuffed my purse with tissue packs just in case I lost the battle with my tears.

Nervous to share the news, I blurted out my prepared script before we even had a chance to order drinks. Then my sweet friend Alex told me how sorry he was to hear this news—that he loved me—and then shared that he had just been diagnosed with HIV. Um, wow. Suddenly, we weren't the only ones in the world dealing with a major health diagnosis. And while you wouldn't wish this kind of thing on a dear friend, his diagnosis made me feel less lonely. He understood what it was to carry the burden of a life-threatening diagnosis. He was navigating his own health care journey while also trying to figure out how (if) to tell those nearest and dearest to him.

We shared with him the disaster of telling our families over the phone before we knew my prognosis. Alex is a communications professional and out of professional habit, he told us he had spent a lot of time since his diagnosis thinking about how to "message" his diagnosis to family and friends. He reminded us that our audience would take its cues from us. If we were upbeat and positive about my prognosis, then our friends and family would be too. "Tell them how to think about it," he advised us. "And oh my God, you're not going to tell everyone *in person* like you are telling me, are you? You're going to exhaust yourselves!"

It was true. The phone calls/texts/emails from our families alone were tough to keep up with. What would we do once that was multiplied by however many friends we told? What he suggested (and what we did) was set up an account on CaringBridge (caringbridge.org). We could then invite friends and family to my personal blog and when there were updates, they would be notified and could read it at their leisure. By centralizing the communication, it would make this one aspect of this ordeal easier. I vowed to start crafting the blog that week.

With my second cancer diagnosis (and fear that there might be more), my opinion that we should keep our communication circle small shifted. I realized I would need to take significant time off from work for all of the treatments I would be undergoing. I also realized that I was going to be bald for a good part of that year, and at that point it would be pretty apparent to everyone that I was battling cancer. In many ways, this just made life easier. I didn't have to worry about who I had told and who I hadn't. It's not like I started announcing it at parties. ("Hi! I'm Sarah and I have cancer.") But I didn't hide it, either. Slowly, I began to accept that cancer was simply part of who I was going to be. At least for now.

I made the controversial decision to *email* a lot of my friends, especially those who lived far away, with the news of both diagnoses. Yes, email. I know this sounds lame, but it really was the most efficient way to get the information out there. Here's what the email I sent looked like:

> *Hello dear, sweet college friends: My apologies that I've been out of touch for awhile -- there's been a lot going on -- and unfortunately, it hasn't been good stuff...My apologies in advance that this is coming in email form -- and not in person -- but I felt it was most important to get the news out...*

In short, I have been diagnosed with cancer...and -- as luck would have it -- two different kinds of cancer! The first one we found is called Adenoid Cystic Carcinoma (ACC is cancer of the salivary gland -- which is really rare) and the other one is breast cancer (which seems like it's frighteningly common). And no, these two cancers aren't related -- apparently I'm just unlucky. :-(The doctors at Stanford are sending me for genetic testing to see if there's a larger story here, but we have our fingers crossed that there is not. The GOOD news (as our doctors have been drilling into our heads) is that both of these cancers are treatable, meaning that surgery and radiation are options for ACC -- and chemo (and surgery and radiation) are options for the breast cancer. I've had the initial surgery to remove the salivary gland cancer -- and this week I will start radiation on my mouth as follow-up to that surgery...also this week I will start chemo to start fighting the breast cancer. Whew. It's a lot, but I am really happy to start getting rid of this disease.

Geoff and I have been trying to get in touch with all of the people we love and let them know what's going on -- and we've set up a website where we will do periodic updates to make it easier to keep everyone in the loop: www. caringbridge.org/visit/sarahbrubachermcdonald.

Anyway -- there's no easy way to tell people you love and don't see often something like this. I'm sorry it's taken me a while to do so -- it's just a tough email to write. I'm happy to talk on the phone or text or email. Sometimes I will be delayed in getting back to you if I have doctors' appts (and I have A LOT of them these days), but I'll do my best. And of course I will have failed to forward this to close friends, so if you see that I'm missing someone (or have the wrong email for someone), please feel free to forward along. I'm a little scattered these

days. :-) Thanks in advance for all of your love and support.
xoxox Sarah

Within 24 hours of sending emails like this, I had a ton of emails/texts/ phone calls to check in. Overwhelming, yes, but also super heartwarming. Folks I hadn't talked to in ages reached out to tell me they loved me. And maybe not as surprising, my people—extended family, friends, co-workers—were super understanding about receiving the news via email and messaged back to tell me how much they appreciated me inviting them to keep tabs via CaringBridge. It made me feel like I had a whole team of folks rooting for me. And I also felt good that the news was out there, relieved that I wasn't hiding anything from anyone anymore.

The email that haunted me in the best possible way during the days/ weeks/months of cancer treatment was from my college friend Hans. I've pasted it below.

From: Hans
To: Sarah
Sent: Sun, March 25, 2012 7:37:30 PM
Subject: your future

Hi Sarah,

I've talked with L's mom. She says that you are whole and healthy and that you are destined to be a wonderful and wise old lady someday.

My guess is that your hair will come in far more beautifully.

G is pretty freaky about this stuff. This is a good sign.

h

My friend Hans is my birthday twin. We met during the first week of college during one of those freshman activity days where there are all kinds of games intended to force awkward first years to meet a ton of people quickly. During the "birthday game," I met Hans as we were the only ones in the basketball gym who shared November 7th as our birthday. Truth be told, I wasn't sure I wanted Hans as my birthday twin. He was intense and hard-driving in a way that I didn't yet recognize as youthful insecurity. I found his intensity overwhelming and didn't have the self-awareness to know that maybe I had a little bit of that intensity myself. With time and confidence, we both mellowed over our four years and became great friends.

After college Hans moved to DC and I moved to NYC. Since both of us were new to the East Coast, we would visit one another every other month to explore our respective cities together. We had a long, comfortable history of overstepping normal boundaries in our candid commentary on one another's lives that only someone who lived through the often-awkward transition from childhood into adulthood with you can get away with.

During one trip to DC, Hans introduced me to a beautiful woman he had just started dating. She was sleek and sophisticated in a greyhound kind of way, with smoothed hair and fitted clothes. I sat next to her at a pub gathering of Hans's work colleagues, but after a dinner of polite conversation that never seemed to spark, I declared to Hans that she was too boring for him to date. Instead, I asked what he thought of Leesa, the woman who was seated across from me at the table. Over beers I had learned she was the first member of her family to move out of the state of Oklahoma *and* the first one to go to college. She was working for a non-governmental organization that was maybe based in Russia. I think she was mastering her fourth language at that point. She was quick, well-informed, and confident without being arrogant. I think she was wearing a flowery skirt and had her hair in a messy bun on the top of her head.

There was none of the sleekness of Hans's current girlfriend but Leesa had *spark*.

Hans's response: "Sarah, Leesa is gorgeous but she's also way out of my league *and* she's a client of mine."

Me: "Well, I think Leesa's amazing. Have you heard her life story? I think you should ask her out. What is the worst that could happen?"

Hans and Leesa were married two years later. God, I love it when I'm right about those things.

Anyway, the amazing Leesa's mother (L's mom) that Hans referred to in his email was a shaman (shawoman?). They have shamen in Oklahoma, apparently. When Hans read my cancer bombshell email, he immediately called his mother-in-law to ask what my outcome would be. She told him I would live to be an old lady. *An old lady*! I knew Leesa's mom couldn't promise this, but the part of me that worried myself awake in the middle of the night just kept reminding myself that a shaman had said I would live. Her words became my talisman.

AUTHOR'S NOTE

Hi there! In the next couple of chapters I will begin the chapter by sharing the 1-2 blog posts I wrote at that point in my cancer treatments. I tried to keep the blog posts pretty newsy and funny where possible (in moments when I could summon a sense of humor). I tried not to dwell on or give too much detail on the roller coaster I was living or the fear I was feeling. It didn't feel helpful to my readers (or to me) to do so at the time. The content you read after the blog posts goes into more detail of what I was really feeling or what I have reflected upon since then. I hope that helps clarify and makes any change in tone (or timeline issues – e.g. Wait, didn't I just read about this in your blog?) less jarring to you as a reader. Thanks!

CHAPTER SEVEN

"SCANXIETY"

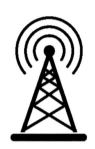

CARINGBRIDGE ENTRY: March 14, 2012

SOME (MUCH NEEDED) GOOD NEWS :-)

Geoff and I met with the Stanford breast oncology and surgery team yesterday. After weeks of what seemed like bad news after bad news, we finally got a break and heard some good news that we wanted to share. At a high level:

Good news:

- All of the extra tests I did (blood, CT, MRI, bone scan) came up clean. The cancer(s) have not metastasized. YAY!!

- My receptors are good. I am estrogen (ER) and progesterone (PR) positive but HER2 (no idea what that stands for) negative. Apparently breast cancer has a whole bunch of subtypes categorized by your receptors. The +/+/- that I have is the most typical subtype and this is really encouraging from a treatment standpoint because after billions of dollars of research, they know what drugs work to kill my specific type of cancer. YAY!

- My breast cancer (actually, both cancers) is slow-growing so we have time on our side to go after it. YAY!

- The doctors think (to be confirmed) they can coordinate the chemo cocktail to allow me to do radiation on my mouth concurrent with the chemo. This is TREMENDOUS news as I had been told we were going to need to focus on the breast OVER the salivary gland and I wasn't crazy about that part knowing that either could recur or spread. It will mean extending the course of chemo, however the tradeoff is totally worth it as it means we can keep treating the ACC. Big YAY.

SO -- a VERY GOOD NEWS day.

Next steps:

- The doctors need to confirm that everyone (both teams) is comfortable with the concurrent treatment plan. We should hear early next week and the plan would be to start treatments immediately.

- I will be doing genetic testing. :-) No one at Stanford has seen these two cancers at the same time (ACC being one of the rarest and breast cancer being one of the most common) and they want to understand if there's a "larger story" (hopefully not).

Thank you ALL for your emails and phone calls and texts. This is going to be a long journey and it is wonderful to have your support and love.

*   *   *

CARINGBRIDGE ENTRY: March 16, 2012

TREATMENT PLAN COMING TOGETHER

The two teams of doctors (head and neck/breast) met yesterday to negotiate my treatment plan to ensure we are fighting the cancers concurrently. I am meeting with the breast oncologist on Monday to finalize the details -- but it will look something like this:

- Phase 1 chemo for the breast - 2x/wk for 12 weeks

- Radiation for the mouth - daily for six weeks (concurrent with chemo)

- Phase 2 chemo continues for another eight weeks - 2x every other week

- Breast surgery

- Radiation for the breast - daily for six weeks

By my calculation, this will mean approximately seven months of bald (five months of chemo -- then maybe two months to grow back in?). I have been gathering opinions from friends who have gone through chemo to determine wig v. scarf. One friend undergoing chemo told me that she felt the scarf made her look too much like a pirate. I thought to myself -- well, I already swear like a sailor -- so maybe the pirate thing isn't so far off... :-)

Regardless of the bald thing, I am REALLY excited that the treatment plan is coming together and that I'll be able to begin fighting shortly. Put me in the game, coach -- I'm ready.

Thank you to all of you for your encouragement. Geoff and I will REALLY need your support as we wade into this. xoxo Sarah

*   *   *

SCANS GALORE

The American Cancer Society says cancer is a genetic "disorder" but that only 5-10% of cancers are thought to be a result of inherited gene mutations. WHAT?! With two confirmed cancers, the Stanford genetics team threw every possible scan and test at me to see if there was a "larger story." Ugh. I had no interest in a larger cancer story. Two cancers were quite enough, thank you. *One* cancer was enough, for that matter. But each time a doctor would suggest a test, I would say *bring on the tests!* I wanted to know what was going on just as much as they did (probably more so).

MRI

When I arrived for my head and neck MRI, I was asked to fill out a form that asked the helpful question, "Are you claustrophobic?" Huh. I narrowed my eyes and thought about that. I was not afraid of elevators but the thought of climbing into a coffin made my palms sweat. I took a deep breath and marked it "no."

My name was called and I followed the nurse down a long hallway of closed doors until we reached a series of dressing rooms. I was asked to change into a hospital gown that tied in the back but which I just knew would gape open to reveal my backside as I walked down the hall with the technician. Foreseeing this awkwardness, they issued me a pair of "one-size-fits-all" pants which clearly were not meant for middle-aged women who like wine and cheese.

Dressed in my MRI uniform, the technician took me into an exam room and put an IV into my arm so that halfway through the MRI they could pump contrast into my veins to get a better image. The technician then led me into a large, antiseptic hospital room with an intimidating machine that had a plastic white tunnel in the middle of it. The air conditioning was on *full blast* in order to keep this gigantic machine cool. In anticipation of my freezing to death, the technician asked if I wanted a *warmed* blanket to be placed on me while I did the test. Oh thank God. Yes. I would like four of them.

There was a pallet sticking out of the tunnel and I was asked to lie face up on the pallet. The technician offered me headphones and/ or earplugs to wear. She said they could pipe classical music into the headphones (which sounded awesome), so being a newbie, I declined the earplugs so I could hear the music better. (Note: *Huge* mistake. The knocking sound that the magnets made drowned out the sound of the music and all I got was a throbbing headache. It was like being too close to the speakers at a concert but without the benefit of, you know, the *music...*)

She handed me a cord with a small plastic bulb at the end of it. This was the panic button. The great news is that if something bad were to happen—like the *big* California earthquake or thermonuclear war or a run-of-the-mill panic attack—I could press the button and (good news!) they'd stop the scan. The bad news was...they'd stop the scan. I knew pressing the panic button wasn't an option for me as I needed the doctor(s) to have the best view of what was going on inside of me. I took a deep breath and told myself to be brave.

The technician patted my leg and then left me alone in that big room to go into her control room. The first thing I heard was, "Okay, we're going to move you into the machine." The pallet I was on started moving and I closed my eyes. My arms bumped against the sides of the tunnel and I began to feel constricted space all around me while I was conveyored into the white tunnel. I thought about that "claustrophobia" question now. This space was small. I tried not to think about how hard it would be for me to wriggle out of it if I needed to. I kept my eyes shut tightly. I didn't want to see how close the top of the tunnel was to my face.

"OK! We're going to get started" I heard the technician say. "We're going to do a total of ten scans. This first one will be four minutes long.

Please don't move." I checked in with my body. Everything seemed to be still except wow, was I breathing hard. Oh God. I needed to slow my breathing so the scan could get a clear picture. But I am in a freaking coffin – how the hell am I supposed to slow my breathing?! But slowly I did and 45 minutes later, I emerged from the tunnel – shaken, but ok.

CT SCAN

A few days later, I had a CT scan (computed tomography scans – also known as a CAT scan). As with the MRI, I donned a drafty gown and tight pants and a technician gave me an IV so he could inject a contrast liquid in me during the scan. This time, as I entered the antiseptic hospital room, I was delighted to find a smaller, less intimidating donut-shaped machine. The technician asked me to lie down face up on a pallet again. I wasn't offered earplugs, headphones, or a panic button. There was no need! The donut was wide and open and the technician assured me he would warn me before each step of the process – including when he would inject the contrast. He warned me that the contrast would make me feel as if I had wet my pants (um... what?) but I shouldn't worry about that. The scan would be completed in less than 15 minutes. This was definitely the scan for me. I sat down and, if possible, I relaxed.

The technician went to his control room and in no time the machine started to hum and "whirl" as it scanned my body. As promised, the technician announced he would be injecting me with the contrast. I felt a slight warmth in my IV arm as the contrast entered my body. I tried to track the warmth as it moved through my bloodstream. And then the funniest thing started to happen. All of the warmth seemed to concentrate itself right there in my crotch. At first I thought maybe I was imagining things, but no, it got super warm. Down there.

Jeez. How warm is this going to get?

And then it was over.

BONE SCAN

The final test the doctors asked me to take was a bone scan. I was told this scan would determine whether there was that whole "larger story" going on—whether possibly one or both of my two cancers had spread to other parts of my body. *Deep breath.*

Like the scan expert I was becoming, I put on the drafty hospital gown and tight hospital pants. I was given an IV – and then (whoa) injected with radioactive stuff (!!!). This technician told me I would need to wait about an hour for the radioactive stuff to make its way through my body.

I was led down to the basement of the building into a room with another huge machine, this one with big arms. I lay down on a pallet and was given instructions to be still while the arms scanned over me like some large photocopy machine. The machine was apparently taking pictures of my bone structure. I was now used to lying still but allowed my eyes to follow the movements of the arms.

After the scan, I joined the technician at his computer. He explained to me that the radioactive stuff they injected me with goes wherever there is a lot of "bone turnover" activity. I wasn't familiar with this concept, but he explained that tumors are effectively a concentration of rapidly reproducing cells. In the bone scan pictures, the places with a lot of activity (tumors) would show up as black on the scan while the bones would show up as light gray. I willed myself to look from the face of the technician to my pictures on his screen.

What I saw was a light gray skeleton. I opened my eyes wider to see if I could see any black spots on the gray. I didn't see any. I asked the technician if he saw anything I wasn't seeing. He said he didn't see anything.

"Does this mean it hasn't spread?" I almost whispered to him.

"It hasn't spread," he told me. For now, there was no "larger story."

GENETIC TESTING

Scans completed, I went back to the genetic team and spoke with the head of the department, Dr. Genetics, about my family history of cancer—which didn't feel to me like it was all that extensive. My grandfather may have had prostate cancer, but he died in his nineties, presumably of old age. My uncle had just died two years earlier from colon cancer, but colon cancer wasn't related to salivary gland cancer or breast cancer. My father had prostate cancer that had recently metastasized, but it also wasn't related to my cancers. On my mother's side there was no cancer at all.

In 2012, they could test five of my genes. None of the women in my family had had cancer, however they still tested me for the BRCA-1 and BRCA-2 suppression genes. (Nope, I didn't have the mutations.) The geneticists also tested me for a gene called TP53 (tumor protein 53). Since I can never remember the name of this gene, I refer to it as the *all-cancer-all-the-time* gene. If I had this mutation, my body's ability to prevent cancer would be severely impacted so it would not be surprising to see multiple developments of cancer. *This* is what the doctors were afraid was going to be my "larger story," but I also tested negative for TP53 mutation.

I asked Dr. Genetics what his theory was: "We have no idea why your body has produced these cancers." Huh.

Dr. Genetics' team took a couple of vials of my blood and told me that as they continue to study cancer, my blood, my genome will be part of those studies. If they figure something out, they'll call me.

As my friend Suzie often reminds me, "Doctors don't know everything. That's why they call it 'practicing medicine.'" :-)

CHAPTER EIGHT

AND SO IT BEGINS

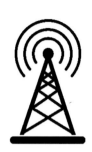

CARINGBRIDGE ENTRY: March 22, 2012

AND SO IT BEGINS...

My friend Suzie joined me yesterday as I met with various doctors and techs to be fitted for all of the gear I will need for chemo and radiation. Because this first round of radiation is to my mouth, they molded a mask to my head which they will use to ensure my head is in the exact same position each time they radiate. I also get a mouthpiece and a specially fitted pillow. The customization experience was not unlike a perverse version of a spa day meets-being-outfitted-as-a-hockey-goalie. Oddly customized to my needs, but I am ready for battle.

Chemo starts Tuesday (3/27). Good news is that it has been adjusted to only once a week. Yipppeee! And I am told that I won't feel bad the day of chemo -- so I can continue to sing in my vocal jazz group Monday nights. This is terrific news.

Radiation starts Wednesday (3/28). Unfortunately, this is every day for six weeks. Ick. But they give free parking. :-)

*Geoff decided we need to get away for a couple of days
prior to starting these treatments -- so we are headed south
down the California coast. Note: I will not be able to drink
wine for five months, so of course the notion of a bender has
been raised...But mostly this weekend will be about hiking
the coast, soaking in hot tubs (also not allowed during
chemo), and breathing through all of this.*

*   *   *

CARINGBRIDGE ENTRY: March 29, 2012

BIG WEEK

Wow -- *now I remember why I have never kept a diary. You
get behind and suddenly you have huge updates to make!
Apologies in advance for the length -- I will try to keep it
organized/concise with headings. Choose your topic. :-)*

BIG SUR: *Let's start with the fun stuff. Geoff and I drove
down to Big Sur on Thursday morning to spend a couple
of days at Ventana Inn & Spa to pamper ourselves before
the treatments began. It was mid-week, so of course they
upgraded us to a suite. The weather was unbelievably
gorgeous -- our room had a hammock (which we napped
in) -- there was on-property hiking with panoramic views of
the Pacific -- two hot tubs to choose from -- a sauna and spa
-- and REALLY good food. Truly -- a perfect getaway. We also
sneaked across the road to the Post Ranch Inn for lunch and
had the joy of whale watching while munching our salads
and sipping our albarinos. :-)*

MONDAY: Port surgery. *On Monday I had a "port" installed
on the right side of my chest. The port is basically this button
thing that is inserted under your skin and into your veins and*

which allows immediate access to your bloodstream. This means when doctors want to do an IV (for chemo, to give anesthesia, to take blood) -- they simply stick a needle into the port instead of doing the whole vein thing. I have to say that this is about the coolest thing/medical advancement I've seen that I didn't know about. Yes, I am a little sore from the surgery -- but I kind of feel like the bionic woman. Happy to show it to you when I see you.

TUESDAY: Chemo. I was pretty nervous about this day as I didn't know how my body would react to the medicine. But since it was my first day -- they gave it to me slowly -- AND because I will be doing radiation concurrently with chemo -- they are giving me low dosages of this particular medicine (taxol). It went pretty quickly and I felt fine afterward (which I am told is typical of the first time). So -- my only side effect of this day was that I woke up the next day a little bit flushed.

WEDNESDAY: Haircut. My hair stylist (and friend) Kathleen recently suggested in her guestbook post that I come in for a short cut to help prepare Geoff and me for the baldness that is coming. So yesterday I cut off my hair and added color. Whoo hooo! I will post photos soon so that you can see it. For those of you who knew me from 1996-98, it is similar to that cut, but not dyed black (for those of you who didn't know me -- these were my badass NYC days). :-)

Radiation: Wednesday was also my first day of radiation (to my mouth). I am told by the nurse that the two minutes they radiate my left mandible area burns 1,800 calories(!!). I am also told that I have no dietary restrictions now (except alcohol) and that I should eat more to keep my weight up. I have never been told to eat more. Wow. I am also given a *litany of mouthwashes and salves to help abate the effects of burning your mouth and face. That part is less fun.*

THURSDAY: *(Today) More radiation -- and now adding a weekly acupuncture appointment to ensure that both the East and West are represented in my healing process. This Eastern part of the healing process I am really looking forward to. It stills my mind and steadies my breathing.*

Thanks to all who made it this far in this long post. Thank you also for all of your love and kindnesses. xoxox Sarah

*   *   *

VENTANA BIG SUR

We headed down to Big Sur for a couple of days to a resort Geoff had heard of called Ventana Big Sur. We hoped we could turn off the cancer channel for a couple of days before the treatments really began.

I was super excited that the doctors had agreed that we could treat both cancers at the same time. I would start radiation to my mouth to zap all of the microscopic ACC cells that might still be in my mouth while I was simultaneously infused with taxol chemotherapy to begin chasing the breast cancer cells that might be floating around in other parts of my body. But I was also scared about the side effects I might experience. Certainly I had heard about the radiation side effects from Dr. HeadNeck (fatigue, dry mouth, mouth sores), and I had read about the side effects of chemo (fatigue, nausea, mouth sores, neuropathy, itchiness, chemo brain...that list seemed endless), but how would *my* body react to each of these? Or rather, *both of these* at the same time? All of that would be revealed in the coming weeks and months, and I just hoped I was up to it.

We pulled into the parking lot and headed into the front desk area. You could smell the clean scent of brush and dirt which surrounded the understated elegance of Ventana. It is one of those resorts that doesn't have a formal check-in desk. Instead, they have an area at the end of this beautiful sunlit room where there are two desks each with a concierge seated behind a computer and two cushy seats in front of the desk for guests to sit as they are checked in. Geoff had called ahead to let the resort know that this was a special visit for us as I was starting my cancer treatments.

As we settled into the seats, the lovely young man who was our concierge started walking us through all of the amenities the resort had to offer and then he looked me in the eye and said, "and Mrs. McDonald, we understand that congratulations are in order on the completion of your cancer treatments."

Unfortunately, I was feeling pretty fragile given my anticipation of how hard the chemo and radiation might be, so tears started rolling down my face. I tried to brush them away as I said in a very soft voice, "Actually, no...I start them next week." The concierge looked at me—stricken—and upgraded us.

We spent three days and nights in a little bungalow that had a king-sized bed, stunning picture windows, a gas fireplace if the temperature dipped, and a large hammock out front. We took long walks, soaked in the Japanese baths, took a yoga class, had a couples massage, and ate anytime food was placed in front of us. I don't know if we even discussed cancer or what lay ahead of us. We just tried to breathe.

MONDAY: PORT SURGERY

I had never heard of a port before the doctors suggested I have one installed to make treatment easier on my veins. I was fascinated by the idea that the medical teams could "plug into" my veins rather than needing to give me an IV every time. Since Dr. BreastOnc had told me that my chemo would take five plus months of weekly treatments, this seemed like a no-brainer to me.

So on a Monday at the end of March, I had a port installed just below my right collarbone and *the day after that* I was good to go for my first chemotherapy session.

TUESDAY: CHEMOTHERAPY

Before I was diagnosed with cancer, I would have probably told you that chemotherapy is a *caustic poison*. This thinking isn't wholly wrong, but it isn't wholly right either. Since diagnosis, I've reframed it for myself. I now think of chemotherapy as a *healing medicine that freaking kills cancer cells*. The way Dr. BreastOnc described it to me, "chemotherapy erases the footprints that cancer may have left in various parts of the body." I really liked that imagery a lot.

Because I was battling *two* cancers that needed to be treated concurrently, the doctors proposed they switch up the typical protocol to allow me to do chemo at the same time as I was receiving radiation to my mouth. Normally, folks with my kind of breast cancer (E+,P+, HER2-) start with A/C (Adriamycin and Cytoxan) followed by a kinder, gentler chemo called Taxol. Since chemo intensifies the effects of radiation, they decided to start with the gentler chemo. *Thank God.*

I arrived at the blood lab an hour prior to my scheduled chemo infusion so they could take some blood (via my port!) and "check my counts." By "checking my counts," the doctors were measuring my red blood cell count, white blood cell count, platelets, and so forth to ensure they were all within normal range. If something like my white blood cells were out of whack, it could indicate my body was fighting an infection and the doctors might decide I should skip chemo that week. This first week I passed with flying colors and was told I could walk on over to the infusion center.

I took a deep breath, walked across the street, up the stairs, and checked in at the desk of the infusion center. On the walls they had TV screens playing videos of mountain streams to calm all of us waiting for our turn.

My name was called and the nurse brought me back to one of the beige pleather La-Z-Boys by the window. She explained that she would be "titrating" my chemo, meaning that she would give it to me slowly to see how I reacted before they opened up the chemo floodgates, so to speak. The nurse started by confirming who I was while she hooked up an IV to my port. The IV was filled with anti-nausea and anti-inflammatory meds to proactively address any "adverse effects" I might have from the chemo. Once my identity was confirmed, she left to order my chemo cocktail from the pharmacy.

I looked around. In my infusion room there were about eight La-Z-Boy chairs. Four were placed at the windows and four were along the walls. (I made a mental note to always grab one by the window.) Each La-Z-Boy had an arm extending from it with a small television so patients could distract themselves with TV if they wanted. Mobile IV units were placed next to the chairs for easy, dedicated access to infusion bags. Finally, each area had additional seats placed next to the chair so that friends and family could sit alongside the patient while the infusion took place.

Geoff set himself up in one of those chairs with his laptop perched on his knees. While my proactive meds pumped into me, Geoff typed away at his computer. You know they say "Til death do us part" when you're getting married but I didn't quite expect that I was going to need to call on Geoff's loyalty to that statement so early into our marriage. And here he was – driving me through thunderstorms and tear storms to every doctor appointment. Holding me as I shared every irrational and rational fear with him. I now needed him in ways I had never anticipated I would ever need anyone. He was my grounding – my touchstone to this physical life. And in the future, he might very well become my nurse and last person I saw if/when I left this physical life. Looking over at him now—balancing working hard for his company while also showing up for his wife—I knew I had chosen the right life partner. I knew I could count on him to be there with me no matter what came.

I mostly looked out the window and thought about the potential side effects I had read about. Would I be nauseated? Would I pass out? What does an allergic reaction feel like? Would I be able to walk out of the infusion center afterward or would I have to be admitted to the hospital? I knew I was playing out the worst-case scenarios, but I was really nervous. I focused on my breathing and tried to relax.

The nurse returned with my IV bags of chemotherapy. There was more confirming of my identity and the type of medication I was to be treated with, and then she attached the first bag of chemo to my IV. As the meds started flowing into my bloodstream, the nurse stood by and watched me. I felt a bit like we were all standing around waiting for me to cliff dive. Here I am standing at the precipice of a huge chemo cliff, and I really didn't want to jump at all—but I knew I *needed* to jump to make myself better. And once I jumped, was I diving into a cool, soothing pool or onto painful rocks? I tried to remind myself that the nurse was there to magically pull me out of the jump if it looked like I was headed for the rocks.

For three hours, we all watched one another and held our collective breath as my body took on the chemo and...nothing happened. When the infusion bags were empty and all of the medicine had gone into my body to begin killing cancer cells, I was excused to go home. Geoff and I picked up our belongings and walked out of the infusion center and to the parking garage. I didn't feel dizzy or in any way weird even though mentally I kept thinking, *Wow, I have chemo in me. Wow.* But that was it. I had survived my first infusion.

WEDNESDAY: RADIATION

On Wednesday, the day after my first chemotherapy infusion session, I had my first radiation session. It was a very busy week. Thursday I planned to rest...and get more radiation. As I understand it, radiation therapy is given every day (except weekends because apparently tumors don't grow on weekends) for 33 days. (Yes, that is a joke.)

The week before my first radiation, I had to meet with a group of technicians to create a mask for me to wear each time I was radiated. The process of creating the mask was super memorable (read: freaky). I was asked to lay on a cot so they could place this *really hot*, wet, meshy fabric over my face. The nurses and I were joking that it was similar to getting a hot towel at a spa but then, oh my freaking God, I didn't expect how *hot* this freaking meshy towel was. I wanted to gasp from the heat, but the technician had warned me to keep my face still while the mask cooled or (like you were warned when you were a kid and making a face, it would stay that way) we'd have to start over again. Luckily, the mask cooled as it hardened and the whole process was over reasonably quickly.

The radiation department was down in the basement of the main medical building because, you know, you'd hate to expose living beings to all of those harmful radiation waves. Ugh. I looked around at the other folks in hospital gowns in the waiting room to try to determine what other kinds of cancer were sitting with me. Most of the folks in the room were older (men who, like my Dad, were getting their prostates zapped?), but there was also one young woman in her twenties who'd had the side of her head shaved. I could see the scar where they must have operated. Ugh. Brain cancer. There were also toys and books for children who might come into the waiting room. I tried to imagine the children were there with their parents who were receiving radiation—that the children themselves weren't there for radiation treatment.

My name was called. I followed the technician into a room with walls that were at least three feet thick. Along the walls there was a large shelving unit where masks and other forms that presumably would keep body parts in place during radiation were kept. In the center of the room was the large radiation machine. And hey! My new mask was already waiting for me on the platform in front of the machine. The technician asked me to lie down and then she placed the mask over my face and snapped me onto the platform. "Alright! This will just take a minute!" she said cheerily and she exited the room, closing the three-foot-thick door with what sounded like a definitive slam.

It was only when she left the room that I suddenly thought: *Wait. Is this going to hurt?* I started to hyperventilate as I thought about the laser beam that was about to be focused on my head. Over a speaker, the technician told me she was about to get started and I started to moan softly to myself.

I glanced out of the mask toward the arm of the machine that was making its way toward me. "Breathe!" I ordered myself. "Calm down. Breathe!" I could see a little red light at the end of it and thought I should close my eyes so as not to look directly at the laser beam while it was making its way across my mask. I ignored my own command to "breathe" and held my breath and listened to the beep-beep-beep of the machine. I braced myself for what I imagined would feel like burning or cutting or stinging. I waited. Beep-Beep-Beep. I checked in with my jaw. Beep-beep-beep. Did it hurt? Nope. It didn't hurt. Beep-beep-beep. I didn't feel anything. After about a minute the beeping stopped and it was over and the technician was back in the room unsnapping me and telling me she'd see me tomorrow. I let out a huge sigh of relief. One down, 32 more sessions to go.

CHAPTER NINE

PREPARING FOR BALD

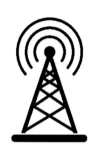

CARINGBRIDGE ENTRY: April 6, 2012

WEEK TWO DOWN

High-level Update: I have just completed week two of my
twenty week treatment plan -- whoo hooo! I've had eight
radiation treatments and two chemotherapy treatments,
and I am happy to report that I'm feeling just fine.

Side effects: Very few so far -- and I am feeling very lucky
about that. I have no fatigue, no nausea, am only starting to
experience mouth sensitivity -- and I still have hair. I would
call that success. The day after chemotherapy my face looks
flushed and I am warm -- but honestly -- the chemotherapy
has been kind to me so far.

Save the Date I: I am told that it's likely my hair will
start falling out in the next two weeks. My hair stylist Kathleen
has kindly offered to host a head-shaving party (yes, this
means you can participate in the shaving of my head) at her
salon in Laurel Heights, and I'm going to take her up on it. We
are currently targeting Wednesday, April 18th for said party

(adult beverages to be served) so if it is convenient for you to join, please plan on doing so. That said -- if my hair does not start falling out prior to April 18th, I'm canceling and pushing it out to May. I may sound all devil-may-care about my hair -- but if I can hold onto it for a couple more weeks -- I'm doing it. ;-) I will post on this blog when/if the party is happening and what the address/time are.

***Save the Date II:** My vocal jazz group is performing April 25th at the St. Francis Yacht Club. I'm still optimistic that I'll be able to sing with them (hair or no hair). If you're interested in attending, lemme know -- we would love for you to join. (They have adult beverages at the yacht club too.)*

***Summary Metrics:** Old habits die hard. It is difficult to go through something like this and not think in terms of what it will take to complete it successfully...So I'm thinking in terms of my treatment metrics and thought I would share them with you:*

Radiation: *30 total sessions/8 completed*   *27% complete*

Chemo I: *12 total sessions/2 completed*   *17% complete*

Chemo II: *8 total sessions/0 completed*   *0% complete*

Total treatment: *20 total weeks/2 completed*   *10% complete*

*Geoff is telling me I'm a freak for sharing these metrics with you, but I know that **so many of you reading this** will enjoy knowing the numbers.*

:-) xoxo Sarah

*   *   *

CARINGBRIDGE ENTRY: April 13, 2012

I STILL HAVE MY HAIR! : -)

Mouth sores appear. *:-(So, after so proudly reporting to all of you for the past two weeks that I wasn›t having any side effects,* **of course** *mouth sores appeared with a vengeance last weekend. Whew! I went on an all-liquid diet (truffle salt is a wonder of this world) and reported the bad news to my doctors on Monday. As a result....*

Chemo was canceled this week. *Turns out that chemo intensifies the radiation. So the doctors conferred and decided to cancel chemo for this week to allow my sores to heal. The doctor is already feeling changes to the tumor in my breast/feels the chemo is working well -- and said it's okay to push out treatment a week. I will be back on a reduced Taxol protocol starting Tuesday.*

Headshaving (re-)scheduled for May 2nd. *Because the chemo gets pushed out a week -- so does retention of my hair. Yeehaw! The* **new** *time/date for head shaving will be 7pm Wednesday, May 2nd. I claim the right to reschedule again should I still have a full head of hair as we near May 2nd. It is unlikely, but humor me.*

What's up with burning 1,800 calories per radiation session? Many interested readers of this blog contacted me to ask how it is that I am burning 1,800 calories per radiation session. So I asked the doctor. Apparently radiation: 1. speeds up the metabolism and 2. creates mouth sores (check), and you burn calories healing mouth sores (!?!). If this is true, I can assure you, jealous readers, that I burned more than 1,800 calories per day this week.

*Summary metrics. Wow, did all of you help me defend my metrics freakishness to Geoff? I received **so many** emails telling me how helpful you found these. Yay -- I'm so very glad. Me too.* ☺

Radiation: *30 total sessions/13 completed -->*	*43% complete (Tuesday will mark 50%)*
Chemo I: *12 total sessions/2 completed -->*	*17% complete (no change)*
Chemo II: *8 total sessions/0 completed -->*	*0% complete*
Total treatment: *20 total weeks/2 completed -->*	*10% complete*

Please note that Tuesday of next week (April 17th) will mark the 50% point for radiation. Whoo hoo! Thanks again for all of the love and support. Xoxo Sarah & Geoff

*   *   *

TIME ALONE

The voices in my head were tough. When I was at home alone, sitting on the couch, the voices in my head whispered fearful things to me. What does the progression of this disease look like? Where will it go next? My lungs? My bones? My brain? Is the cancer spreading in my body as I sit here? Once cancer has spread, can it be reversed? I am in stage 3 for breast cancer—what does stage 4 look like? Does anyone ever survive stage 4? What *can* the doctors do? How painful will the cancer (and the treatments) be? Will I spend days/weeks/months getting sicker and sicker? What does "sick" look like for me? Will I be able to go out and be with people, or will I be confined to our apartment and my bed—quarantined due to fear of exposure to others—for fear that I will get an infection my exhausted body won't be able to fight? Will I lose control of my functions—my stomach, my bowels, my brain? Will I be able to maintain my dignity as I slowly lose control of my bodily functions? Will I need to confine myself to our apartment because I won't be able to trust that I can control my body when I am with others—slowly and steadily reducing my orbit until I am alone in my bed enduring each indignity given to me by this relentless disease?

Will I be alive a year from now?

Ultimately I was alone, waiting. I am sitting here on the couch waiting to find out what happens next. I am waiting to hear what the tests and scans tell us. I am waiting to hear what treatments the doctors will suggest. I fear I am waiting for my death.

Surrounded by other living beings, I am lonely. I am on Cancer Island, cut off and remote. I stop buying new clothes because I don't trust I will be alive in a year to wear them and their purchase seems frivolous and naively optimistic. The people around me are troubled by work, by the news, by social media, by other trivial things that consume them. How is it that a few short weeks ago I could be kept up at night by something as insignificant as my work to-do list? How did that ever seem important? My to-do list has been reduced to "live."

I have Geoff. I have friends who take walks with me or meet for lunch, who bring me food, who text and email and call. I have people who are helping me fill up the waiting hours with activities. But ultimately, I am alone in facing this disease. When the doctors are telling me what they see in the scans, they are speaking to me, alone. While Geoff can hold my hand, it is me alone who receives the chemotherapy, the radiation, the surgery.

I cannot share the voices in my head with them, not even with Geoff. Out loud, my voices sound pitiful and overdramatic. I am embarrassed and muted by them. I fear losing my composure if I speak of them, of losing all control of my emotions, of losing my dignity.

Very unhelpfully, as I sit on my couch, I do what I know I shouldn't do. I google the statistics—the survival rates for my cancers. I am told that for my breast cancer, the average five-year survival rate is 90%. The average 10-year survival rate is 83%. I can get behind these numbers. I can will myself to believe that I will be included in those large survival numbers. With those statistics, I can muffle the voice in my head that tells me I will die of breast cancer.

The statistics for the salivary gland cancer are harder, and it is Dr. Maxillofacial's voice I hear when I read them. The internet tells me that "although most patients with ACC are alive at 5 years, a majority of patients die from their disease 5 to 20 years after diagnosis." Also, "adenoid cystic carcinoma (ACC) is an aggressive, often indolent tumor, with a high incidence of distant metastasis (DM)." The words "relentless" and "incurable" are peppered throughout the summaries I read.

I try to remind myself that "incurable" and "terminal" are not the same words.

GUIDED IMAGERY

I wish I could find the exchange of texts I had with Dr. Fertility from that first weekend on Cancer Island. Dr. Fertility is one of those unbelievably qualified people you hear about who also happens to be just unimaginably thoughtful and kind. She texted me on that first Saturday after diagnosis to see how I was doing and I responded honestly: that I was f***ing freaked out. She said she wasn't sure how open I might be to the idea, but that she really believed in the linkages between mind and body, and that I might consider exploring "guided imagery" as a therapy to help me come to terms with my diagnosis. A quick Google search on guided imagery indicated that it was "a form of focused relaxation that helps create harmony between the mind and body. It is a way of focusing your imagination to create calm, peaceful images in your mind, thereby providing a 'mental escape.'" Hmm. This sounded like meditation.

Prior to my cancer diagnosis, I had attended exactly two yoga classes (with meditation) because my friend Tripti had *asked* me to attend the class. She had just begun studying to be a yoga instructor and was teaching classes on Monday nights at a studio convenient to my nightly drive home. However, "convenient to my nightly drive home" didn't exactly translate for me into "interested in attending." Tripti's yoga class began with 10 minutes of meditation. Both times I attended I found myself sneaking glances at the clock. 7:02. 7:05. Ugh—only 7:08!? *When will this freaking class end*!? I didn't feel like I had time to "waste" at a yoga class, meditating. I had *things to do*. This whole guided imagery thing sounded like *meditation-with-words* which might actually be worse than *yoga-with-meditation*.

I scrolled down to the first website listed in my guided imagery Google search —Health Journeys. I found Health Journeys had 27 (!) different categories for which they had a guided imagery audio file. "Cancer" was listed as a category, but so was depression, hospice & palliative care, illnesses & conditions, and mental & emotional health. And that was just the first column of categories. Mentally, I took note in the event I needed any of these other categories as I progressed in my cancer treatments.

I decided to *GO BIG*. There was a box set of guided imagery CDs dedicated to helping navigate cancer. The CDs included "Fight Cancer," "Relieve Stress," "Chemotherapy," and "General Wellness." I bought the bundle and waited for them to arrive.

On the day the CDs arrived, I opened the "Relieve Stress" CD, popped it into my laptop's drive, and put on my headphones. The tips & tricks section on the website had told me that any time of the day worked to listen to the CDs, though they suggested you choose a time you didn't expect to be interrupted. (I closed the bedroom door.) I should sit in a comfortable place (at the foot of my bed, back against the bed). It also assured me that "You do not have to be a 'believer' for it to work. Positive expectancy helps, but even a skeptical willingness to give it a try is enough." Okay—that was a good thing because I was plenty skeptical.

Feeling kind of silly, I scooched into my seated position, closed my eyes, and hit play. At first I heard instrumental soothing music. Then a voice that was low and calm started speaking. I couldn't help thinking as she spoke, *Is this voice annoying? I don't think so. Do I like this voice? Maybe. Wait. What is she saying?* And then I started to listen.

The voice was encouraging me to walk in my mind's eye to a place I loved and to look around—see the grass or the water or the trees, feel the breeze. There then ensued an extended argument within my brain as to *which* place I should choose. Should it be somewhere I go regularly? Where I run or hike? Or should it be somewhere significant from my childhood? Oh for Christ's sake, just *choose something,* I'm falling behind on this guided walk! I settled on the walk through the white birch trees between Bay Beach and Slim Point at Silver Bay, New York—a place from my childhood.

I walked from the grassy patches of Bay Beach down to the rutted walkway that leads into the forest of white birches. I walked into the birches and there, among the imagined trees, I started crying. This was not the kind of crying where gentle, sweet tears run down my face. This was the wracking, snot-releasing sob of crying where animal sounds escape from your throat. I could not remain seated against the bed. I had to get up on my knees and then lean over to allow the sobs to work their way through me. I stayed in this prone position—what I would later learn was "child's pose" from Tripti—listening and crying, until the CD ended. Crying because I didn't know what the next year would hold. Crying because I was so scared. Crying because I felt so helpless and oftentimes, hopeless. Crying in the safety of my bedroom with the door closed, huddled into a fetal position. Because even though I knew my husband and my family and my friends were all on the other side of the door, I also knew that when it came down to it, it was going to be me and this cancer doing our dance. I would be alone on that rutted pathway into the white birch trees.

I have no idea why or how this guided-imagery-meditation-with-words worked, but wow, was it the catharsis I needed. I listened to that CD every day, sometimes twice a day, for about two months. And each time I cried. Alone. On my knees. Doubled over. Until one day...the stress released. I didn't wake up with my body tensed and my brain racing to figure out how to escape. Some kind of mind-body magic happened and I just relaxed. I had two unrelated cancers, an uncertain prognosis, and a year of cancer treatments staring me down—but at least now I didn't have the I'm-so-stressed-that-I-might-die-from-a-heart-attack-first at the top of that list.

PREPARING FOR BALD

My oncologist told me that two weeks into chemotherapy I would lose my hair. It would fall out in clumps into the shower drain, onto my pillow, into my hands if I ran my hand through my hair. I made an appointment to cut my shoulder-length hair above the ears short as I had in my early twenties when I was living in New York City. I was twenty-something in the '90s and as I gained short hair confidence, I started going down to the East Village to get my hair cut and *shaved* in the back. I also started dying it black. Despite the shaved black hair, I still wore a suit every day to work with stockings and heels. I saved the combat boots for the weekends.

I liked the new haircut Kathleen gave me, but wasn't convinced it would really prepare me for being bald. A woman from Tripti's yoga class gave me an expensive blonde wig from her own cancer-treatment-bald days, but I kept it in the box – afraid of how familiar I would likely become with it. My brother started shaving his head in his early twenties when his hair started thinning, but that seemed common and acceptable for a man. A bald woman seemed to say only one thing: I have cancer.

My girlfriend Kara invited me over to her home for dinner and to meet her new roommate, Cece. Cece had been struggling with ovarian cancer for a number of years, and she offered to teach me how to wear headscarves. I put on my big girl pants and went over to Kara's on the appointed day. Cece brought out a number of long, cotton swathes of fabric and showed me how to wrap them around my head and into an attractive knot. Cece looked exotic and beautiful in the headscarves. I looked at myself in one of Cece's headscarves and all I could think was: I have cancer.

All of this preparing to be bald was tough...and embarrassing. When you're dealing with the meta-issue of life and death, it feels like being bald should be the least of your worries. It feels petty. It feels vain. But this is the thing—being bald is so public. There's no hiding the *big thing* going on in your life when everyone can see that you're bald. I didn't want people on the street, at the store, or at a restaurant looking at me / pointing at me and saying: She has cancer.

In the meantime, I waited for my hair to fall out.

CHEMO AND DRINKING

I had heard that patients shouldn't drink while they are receiving chemotherapy treatment. I checked in with Dr. BreastOnc about this because I was still enjoying my nightly glass of wine. I asked her if alcohol impacts the efficacy of the chemotherapy and if for that reason I should stop drinking it. She told me the reason doctors advise patients not to drink during chemo is because the liver is already working so hard to process the chemo that adding alcohol can be super taxing for the liver. Also, at some point, most patients lose interest in alcohol because the taste of it changes. I asked if it was okay to continue to drink a glass (or two) of wine a night as long as my weekly blood tests looked good and I still had my sense of taste. Dr. BreastOnc told me she would monitor my liver function weekly and would let me know if she saw an issue.

Hot damn—I could keep drinking!

MOUTH SORES AND METRICS

Toward the end of my second week of radiation, I took the mouthpiece I wore during radiation out of my mouth and there was blood on it. There were multiple sores along my gums and two were beginning to appear on the left floor of my mouth.

"Oh," the technician said as I showed it to him.

"Is that normal?" I asked. "I have some sores that have cropped up in my mouth that must be bleeding."

"Yup, normal to have sores and some bleeding—though we don't usually see them until the end of a patient's radiation protocol. Maybe in the fifth or sixth week. You're only finishing your second week."

I went to get my blood drawn and then on to my oncologist appointment to get approval to take chemo that week. The mouth sores were deemed "toxic" and I was told I would be skipping chemo that week to give my mouth a break. Initially, I was hopeful that when the oncologist said "canceled" it meant that I got to skip that chemo session entirely. Just take it off the table! Um, yeah. Not so fast. What "canceled" meant for me is that the chemo session got pushed out a week and along with it, my completion date.

For a goal-oriented person, it is difficult to have a completion date pushed out. I had been focused on how many radiation sessions I needed to do, and how many chemo sessions I needed to do, and projected that onto my calendar to determine when I would be finished with each of my treatments. At work, I was accustomed to setting up key performance indicators (KPIs) or just plain old metrics to determine whether we were making progress in specific target areas. I decided to do the same with my cancer with those KPIs at the end of each blog entry I called summary metrics. But wow, it was tough when I felt like I was making progress in an area like chemo (two sessions down, only ten to go!) to then have to push that out a week or two. It made me feel like the treatments would never be finished.

CHAPTER TEN

LITE BRIGHT: ADVENTURES IN RADIATION THERAPY

CARINGBRIDGE ENTRY: April 22, 2012

RADIATION IS OVER 50% COMPLETE

BIG NEWS: Radiation is over 50% complete!!! *In fact, as of Friday, it is 60% complete -- or 3/5 complete if you prefer fractions. The good news is the mouth sores went away when I skipped a week of chemo (yay!) -- but then I did a 50% dose of chemo this week and they're back (boo!). But happily -- the end of radiation is in sight (May 8th)...and then I will just be focused on chemotherapy.*

Hmmm...What is all of that hair doing in the shower drain? *So apparently we will be keeping the May 2nd head-shave date. And likely I will look pretty mangey by then as the hair is coming out by the handfuls -- BUT that should only make it more fun. If you're game, I'll see you at 7pm Wednesday,*

Summary metrics.

> ***Radiation:*** *30 total sessions/*
> *18 completed -->   60% complete!!!!*

Chemo I: 12 total sessions/
3 completed -->   25% complete
Chemo II: 8 total sessions/
0 completed -->   0% complete
Total treatment: 20 total
weeks/4 completed -->   20% complete

Thanks again for all of the love and support. Xoxo Sarah & Geoff

*   *   *

CARINGBRIDGE ENTRY: April 30, 2012

HEADSHAVE PARTY POSTPONED

*I am so sorry to be behind on my weekly post for the second week in a row. But...it is for the very best reasons... Last week, my sister visited and walked in my shoes with me for radiation treatments, acupuncture, yoga.☺ This week, my parents were in town. They arrived Wednesday to catch my jazz concert (**and** for the maiden voyage of the BLONDE WIG) and left Sunday morning. It has been busy!*

I STILL have hair(!!) and, in fact, more hair than some close family members of mine. ☺ But this means that, as promised, I'm going to postpone the HeadShaveParty – again. My apologies for any inconvenience this might cause – but I want to hold onto this stuff for as long as I can.

Radiation is 4/5 complete! Whoo hooo! ☺ This is the really big news this week. I am in the single-digit countdown. I only have six more sessions to go and I will be finished with radiation to the mouth and these dumb mouth/throat sores. I could NOT be more excited. The doctor checked my breast tumor today and told me it has "objectively reduced"!! She is super pleased with how well the chemo is going, so she is excusing me from chemo again this week to help get the sores back in line (bless her).

Summary metrics. *It is fun to see the progress!!*

> **Radiation:** *30 total sessions/ 24 completed -->*　　　　　　*80% complete!!!!*
>
> **Chemo I:** *12 total sessions/ 4 completed -->*　　　　　　*33% complete*
>
> **Chemo II:** *8 total sessions/ 0 completed -->*　　　　　　*0% complete*
>
> **Total treatment:** *20 total weeks/5 completed -->*　　　　　　*25% complete*

Thanks again for all of the love and support. Xoxo Sarah & Geoff

*　　*　　*

RUNNING ON THE BEACH

It is one of the many embarrassments of riches to living in San Francisco that I could go running next to the water. To be super clear, I do not love running. Running is uncomfortable for me. I don't lithely glide along the path like a gazelle feeling energized and at one with the larger universe when I run. Running is an effort for me. I am not built as a runner. I am from German farm stock. If running, I should be running after cows needing milking. I should be out tilling the fields and birthing the babies. I do not scamper. I lumber. I gasp for breath. I jiggle where I know a body should not jiggle. But I have found running to be one of the most efficient modes of exercise *and* I get to do it outside. Outside is big for me, so I run outside. Over the past number of years I have taken to running down at Crissy Field, which is right there on the water in front of the Golden Gate Bridge.

I stretched out next to my car in the parking lot. I gave my legs and knees and hips a pep talk, reminding them that when the run was over, they would be really happy. Because it would be over and I wouldn't ask much of them until tomorrow when we would do it again. I finally convinced myself that it was not going to get any warmer and I began my slow lumber toward the running path along the water. Half a mile into the run, there was an opportunity to keep running straight on the path or to take a sharp right to the beach (the road less traveled?). I took the right.

It turned out that it was harder to run on sand than on a compacted dirt running path. I told myself that choosing the beach made my running even more efficient. I promised my legs they wouldn't have to run as far to burn as many calories or work their muscles. But I secretly knew I was lying and I'd still make myself run all the way to the bridge and back anyway. My lumber became even less elegant as I propelled myself forward along the shoreline. I loved running on the beach because I had a better view of the Golden Gate Bridge and the bay and only occasionally had to move quickly sideways up the beach to avoid a wave. There were also very few people running on the beach—so my labored breathing and bad running form were known only to me and the dog walkers who also preferred the shore to the path.

When I got back to the car, I grabbed my workout bag and headed into the sailing club we belong to to use the showers. I removed my sweaty clothes and jumped into the locker room shower. They're pretty utilitarian showers; not meant to pamper so much as to rinse off salt water from chilled female sailors. Since I was actually still sweating, I kept the water on a pretty chilly temp to help cool me down. I stood under the shower head and let it pour all over me. I turned the shower off to conserve water (we're in a drought, California!), squirted shampoo into my hands, and worked it into a lather in my hair. I soaped myself down and then turned the shower back on to rinse everything off. As I was rinsing, I glanced down at the drain.

The drain was completely clogged with hair. *My* hair. Oh God.

I felt my head. I felt hair. I didn't feel bald patches.

I dried off as quickly as I could and got out of the shower and in front of the mirrors. Thankfully no one else was in the locker room at 10:00 am on a Tuesday, so I could examine my head about an inch from the full-length mirrors on my left and right. I seemed to have only lost some of my hair and not in clumps as had been promised—but maybe this was just the beginning.

Nope. Cutting my hair short did not prepare me for this.

SUSAN'S VISIT

I invited my sister to come visit. She arrived on day 15 of radiation. I warned her that it would be halfway through my radiation treatments and four into my chemo treatments, and there was a chance I wouldn't be able to speak due to the sores in my mouth and on my tongue and in my throat. She came anyway.

She spent the week shadowing me. She watched me run on the beach while she drank coffee and listened to the waves. We drove to and from Stanford for radiation sessions. She sat with me during the oncology visits. She waited for them to take my blood. She joined me when I drove all the way to Half Moon Bay just to walk on Gray Seal Beach. She donned a pair of my yoga pants (her first?) and joined me at Tripti's Friday morning yoga class which I was now regularly attending.

LOVING-KINDNESS MEDITATION

After class, Tripti decided to join Susan and me on our drive down to Stanford for radiation. As Susan drove, I shared with them the story of my first radiation session and *how terrified* I had been when the technician strapped me into my mask—so much so that I had begun hyperventilating.

Tripti asked what I was thinking about during the radiation session, and I told her that I was singularly thinking about the motherf***ing laser beam that was about to radiate me. Tripti—who is not a big swearer herself but tolerates my swearing—smiled at me and then gently suggested I try a "loving-kindness meditation" while I was in the radiation mask to both distract and calm me, as well as to send that loving-kindness vibe out into The Universe.

"In a loving-kindness meditation, you might whisper or chant to yourself: May I be well. May I be happy. May I find peace."

"Okay," I said. "So while I'm lying there with the motherf***ing laser pointed at my head, I should internally say to myself: I will be well. I will be happy. I will find peace."

"Um...no. That's not what I said," she said patiently to me. "You don't want to be bossy with The Universe and demand that you be healthy and happy and peaceful. Instead, you want to ask for these things from The Universe. You want to send these loving-kindnesses out into The Universe by saying 'May I...' and not 'I will...'"

"Oh. Okay. Less bossy. 'May I be well. May I be happy. May I find peace,'" I repeated back to her, a little embarrassed by my apparent lack of manners with The Universe.

"Yes, and then once you have sent these thoughts out to The Universe and have established this kind of forcefield of loving-kindness around yourself, you may want to extend the loving-kindness to other people you know who might need this, like your Dad, by saying: 'May *Dad* be well. May *Dad* be happy. May *Dad* find peace.'"

"Oh wow, so I can ask these things of The Universe for other people as well?" I wasn't sure whether I was going to be capable of thinking all of these things while I had a laser beam aimed at my head, but I liked the idea of aggregating my "asks" of The Universe all at one time. It seemed efficient.

"Yes," Tripti said. "And then once you've extended the loving-kindness to your Dad and any others who you know are hurting or need this loving-kindness from your heart, you may want to extend the loving-kindness to all beings in The Universe in the form of something like: May *all beings* be well. May *all beings* be happy. May *all beings* find peace."

She checked my face to see if I was absorbing all of this, whether I was taking it seriously, and whether I could do this without bossing around The Universe. One look at overwhelmed me and she said, "You know what? You don't have to do all of this on your first day of loving-kindness meditation. It will be enough to ask for these things for yourself this first time and work up to asking for it for other people and then The Greater Universe when you have become more comfortable in this practice. Just don't be bossy. It isn't nice, and remember, this is a loving-kindness meditation. It is about loving *and* kindness."

Later, as I lay down on the radiation bay and was strapped into my mask by the technician, I closed my eyes and started thinking of the chant: "May I be well. May I be happy. May I find peace."

I knew I couldn't mouth the chant aloud because the doctors were counting on me to keep everything related to my head still to ensure they radiated the same area every time. Instead, I chanted it inside my head: "May I be well. May I be happy. May I find peace."

Naively, I had thought it would be easy for me to say that chant and then easily extend it to other people—and ultimately all beings in The Universe—on that first day. I mean, it was only a chant, right? It was just words, right? And they were pretty simple, easy-to-remember words.

Except that they weren't simple or easy to remember once I was strapped into the mask, anticipating the laser beam. "Wait...what is the beginning part of the chant? Am I asking for health first or is it peace? And wait, how do I ask without being bossy? Am I being bossy? What was it I said when I was bossy? And what if I just *am* bossy and that's the way it is? If

I'm bossy, does this still work? Does The Universe listen to me if I don't say it in the right order or use the wrong words?" Whew. Somehow all of this "easy" was picking up a whole lot of "complicated" steam and I was really working myself up.

GODDAMMIT, WHY ISN'T THIS EASY!? WHY CAN'T THIS ONE THING BE EASY!?

I stopped. I decided to go back to the beginning. What was the first thing Tripti had told me to say? "May I be well." Yes, I could say that. In fact, I could say that a whole bunch of times: "May I be well. May I be well. May I be well."

Then I decided that for this first day, I would just do my best and just try to ask for what I needed. What else did I need?

"May I be well. May I be healthy. May I be free of cancer.
May I be happy. May I laugh. May I find joy.
May I find peace. May I find peace. May I find peace."

As I said all of these things in my mind, I started to focus on what I was thinking rather than what I was doing. I started to slow my breathing. I started to relax.

"May I be well. May I be happy. May I find peace."
"May I be well. May I be happy. May I find peace."
"May I be well. May I be happy. May I find peace."

I was surprised to hear the technician open the three-foot-wide door and walk over in her squeaky, matte-black clogs to the machine I was strapped into. The radiation session was over. She was telling me it was time to go home.

The next session I was able to get into the groove of the chant sooner—slow my breath and relax—and then extend this loving-kindness mantra to my Dad and to the greater Universe. That loving-kindness meditation, that chant, got me through the remaining rounds of radiation to my head and the subsequent 30 rounds of radiation to my breast the following January and February. It was freaking *awesome*.

Is it why I got better? I honestly don't know. I will tell you the relaxation that chant brought me soothed me in a way the medical statistics did not. It brought a structure and a focus to the radiation sessions that helped me live through them in a serene state of mind rather than the frenzied alarm of my first session. It made radiation easier, and frankly, that is what I needed.

WE EACH GET TO CHOOSE

Cancer is not new to my immediate family. I mean, we're not experts or anything, but we had our introduction to cancer in 2001 when my Dad was diagnosed with prostate cancer. I have heard that if men live long enough, nearly all will be diagnosed with prostate cancer, but that they will likely die from something else because prostate cancer is so slow-growing. But Dad was 63. He wasn't old enough to ignore it, and the treatments available then had obnoxious side effects.

In 2001, the options for prostate cancer patients were:

- **Surgery** to remove the prostate. Possible side effects were incontinence and impotence. Dad wasn't really interested in pursuing a treatment that might result in him wearing diapers, so he did not want surgery. I didn't even touch the topic of impotence with him.

- **Radiation** to kill the cancer cells. We were told side effects would likely be minimal, but in radiating the area, Dad would be removing the option of surgery later as the prostate would be pulverized by the radiation.

- **Do nothing.** In my conversations with him, Dad really wanted to pursue this option as he wasn't feeling any symptoms of the cancer, but he also didn't want it to spread.

Dad spoke with a number of doctors and the prevailing wisdom was that he should pursue the radiation. So in the fall of 2001, Dad went every day for 33 sessions to get his prostate "zapped." (I shamelessly adopted the term "zapping" for my own.) He had no side effects, never felt ill, was really upbeat about the whole thing—and believed he had left this whole cancer thing behind him.

During the holidays of 2010—six months after our wedding—my side of the family gathered at Geoff's and my condo in San Francisco. The weather in San Francisco was typical for that time of year, foggy with a pretty serious chill in the air. Most of us bundled up with fleece and socks, including Dad, but he kept telling me how cold he was. He didn't seem to be coming down with a cold or flu, he was just cold! I suggested he wear my heating pad directly on his chest while he was in the house because my theory was that if he could just heat up his core, he would warm up. But even the heating pad wasn't working. As Mom and Dad got into the car to drive back down to Southern California, I suggested that Dad go see his doctor. When he did, the doctor told him the prostate cancer had returned.

A year after Dad's recurrence, I called to tell him I had cancer. His first worry was that somehow he had given it to me. I assured him that in the case of my adenoid cystic carcinoma, it's not genetic, and in the case of my breast cancer, I didn't have the mutated genes (BRCA1 and BRCA2). Certainly, my genes were mutating, but heredity didn't seem to be playing a role in it. Dad and I had just happened to both get lucky.

Mom and Dad came to visit me the week after Susan visited. I invited them both to join me for a trip to the radiation clinic. Mom was enthusiastic about joining for the scientific fascination of it (read: biology professor). Dad decided he'd already experienced radiation and didn't need the refresher course. Just like I had with Susan, I took Mom to Tripti's yoga class in the morning and then we continued on down to Stanford to the radiation clinic. After radiation, we picked up Dad so we could drive to Sam's Chowder House in Half Moon Bay. As the three of us sat with our bowls of chowder, we talked about the unavoidable: cancer.

At this point, Dad was having trouble walking and needed to rely on a walker to get around, which is a bummer at any age, much less at a young 74. His doctor wanted him to try chemotherapy to slow the spread of the cancer to other parts of his body. I had been doing Taxol for about a month at that point without any really bad side effects (except the hair-in-the-drain situation), so I was a big proponent of Dad doing chemo and halting that cancer. Dad was concerned that chemo would lead to hair loss, and (so far) he had been very private about his cancer. In fact, he had asked that none of us speak with people outside of our immediate family about it. He feared that being bald would make his cancer obvious to everyone (boy, did that resonate with me). I tried to gently ask Dad what was more important, extending/saving his life, or not being bald so folks didn't suspect cancer?

Dad shared a conversation he had just had with his doctor. The doctor asked how he was feeling on a scale of 1-10. Dad had said 4 and then asked his doctor when he could expect to be at 9 or 10 again. "I'm not sure we can get you to 9 or 10 again, Paul. I can maybe get you to 6 but I don't think, given the progression of your disease, that you will be at 9 or 10 again." Dad then asked me if life was worth living if you were only ever at a 4.

He worried aloud about the side effects of chemo—how it would make him feel? Would he be nauseated? How long would he have to do the chemo? Would he have to do chemo for the rest of his life and/or for as long as he wanted to live? Smiling sheepishly, Dad admitted a reason he could see extending his life was in order to see another winning University of Michigan football season.

What!?

I honestly wanted to scream at my Dad that doing chemotherapy shouldn't even be a question. *Of course* he should do chemo—*anything* it would take to extend, or better yet, save his life. But that was my own point of view informed by my selfish need to have my Dad around.

"I can't tell you what to do, Dad. I want you to do chemo, but that's because I'm afraid of losing you. But I also don't want you to be miserable. You need to choose what is best for you."

I realized then—and have thought a lot about this since—that no matter how much I wanted my Dad to do chemo so that he could be around *for me*—whether he chose to pursue treatment or not, was ultimately his decision. Dad got to choose what was best for him. I didn't get to choose for him. And he didn't get to choose for me.

CHAPTER ELEVEN

MOUTH SORES ARE STUPID AND THEY SUCK

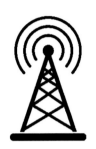

CARINGBRIDGE ENTRY: May 11, 2012

MOUTH RADIATION IS COMPLETE.

Let the mouth sores heal and the eating begin! *Of course you all know how excited I will be to eat again. I'm hoping for the mouth sores to heal sometime early next week. For now, I am on pain meds and am plugging along -- but there is only so much soup/oatmeal/liquid a person can stand -- even if you do add truffle salt. The thing I have missed most? Crunchy vegetables. I am going to have the biggest salad ever once I can stand all of those vegetables poking into the recesses of my mouth. I sound like such a Northern Californian, don't I? Maybe I should have said I crave an organic, locally-sourced, hand-torn, artisan salad.*

So -- what does this mean? What's next? Are you cancer-free in your mouth? *Well, I hope so. I had the surgery in February to remove the salivary gland tumor and now, via* radiation, have now burned every living cell in the left side of my mouth (hence the mouth sores) in the hopes that any pesky cancer cells remaining are destroyed. Next, the doctors will have me do a baseline MRI -- and then an MRI every six months after that (for five years) to ensure the tumor isn't growing back. And that's the story with the ACC -- we will just continue to monitor.

So -- how will you celebrate this end-of-mouth-radiation milestone? Geoff and I are going to spend a day at Indian Springs Resort and Spa in Calistoga. I've never had a mud bath and I hear that mineral springs are healing -- so that's our destination. Hooray!!

Now my cancer treatments will be focused on fighting the breast cancer with chemotherapy. The great news is that even with only four chemo treatments so far, the breast tumor and lymph nodes have started to reduce. Unfortunately, I have 13-16 weeks of chemo ahead -- but it is GREAT to have early indications of success.

Summary metrics. ONE MILESTONE COMPLETED!!!!

Radiation: 30 total sessions/
30 completed -->   100% complete!!!!

Chemo I: 12 total sessions/
4 completed -->   33% complete   No change

Chemo II: 8 total sessions/
0 completed -->   0% complete   No change

Total treatment: 20 total
weeks/7 completed -->   35% complete

Thanks for all of your love and support. Xoxo Sarah & Geoff

*   *   *

CARINGBRIDGE ENTRY: May 21, 2012

MOUTH SORES ARE STUPID AND THEY SUCK.

Antibiotics will hopefully do the trick. *You will remember that I finished radiation May 8th, which is roughly 13 days ago! Plenty o' time for these dumb old mouth sores to take pity on a solid-food-starved person and heal, however they are apparently not playing by my timeline. As a result, today my doctor -- suspecting an infection -- has put me on antibiotics. I have my fingers and toes crossed (and would cross my tongue if I could actually move it) that they will clear this up. The doctor also decided to push chemo out another week to allow my mouth to heal. The only bummer with that is...*

"Skipping chemo" actually translates into "you do chemo longer." *I was pretty psyched when my doctor first had me "skip" a chemo session. We skipped because my mouth sores were bad -- and yet my tumor continued to shrink anyway! Whoo hoo! Naively, I hoped I could conquer this tumor with reduced chemo and still stay on the timeline I had told myself would have me finished with chemo by the end of August. Apparently not. "Skipping" actually means that each time we skip a session, we tack a session on to the end. (People who grew up with snow days might be familiar with this concept.) Yes, I know I didn't delete sessions in my metrics -- but I really was hopeful that "skipping" meant "skipping". GAH.*

Reducing updates from weekly to milestone-driven. *Now that radiation is over, I have reduced my trips to Stanford from daily to 1-2 times a week. To date, I've been giving you weekly updates because the metrics (and the stories) were changing appreciably. I think things will slow down now, so I am going to adjust my updates from weekly to* *milestone-driven. When there's something to report on, you'll hear from me. (Like honestly, you might hear from me when I finally eat that crunchy salad or have a piece of crusty bread. Did I mention I am SOLID FOOD-STARVED? Please feel pity for Geoff.)*

You can sign up for email or text alerts on CaringBridge. *A number of you have asked how you can know when I've posted a journal entry. CaringBridge actually has the functionality where you can sign up for email or text alerts when there is a new post. On the journal page, the word "Notifications" appears in the upper-left corner in purple just under the word "Journal". If you click on "Notifications," you can choose to be contacted via email or text when there is a new post. This is likely a lot easier than visiting the site periodically.*

Summary metrics.

* **Radiation:** 30 total sessions/ 30 completed -->   *100% complete!!!!*
* **Chemo I:** 12 total sessions/ 5 completed -->   *42% complete*
* **Chemo II:** 8 total sessions/ 0 completed -->   *0% complete   No change*
* **Total treatment:** 20 total weeks/8 completed -->   *40% complete*

Thanks for all of your love and support. Xoxo Sarah & Geoff

*   *   *

APEX OF THE PAIN

I was really excited for our celebration day at Indian Springs. I had read they had mud baths—which I had never done before—and it just sounded like one of those quintessential Northern California things I needed to do. Geoff assured me that Indian Springs had these great midweek packages available where we could have a mud bath, followed by the steam room, followed by full-body massage *plus* all-day access to their hot springs (!!) all for a "reasonable" cost. Geoff asked for the day off and I started looking forward to our day together *and* the end of radiation.

At the end of week two, I had sores and some bleeding, so you have to believe that by the end of week six, the situation in my mouth was bleak. You know when you bite your lip and then keep accidentally biting it for the next five days? Well, it was like having fifteen of those all below my tongue, on the inner part of my jaw, and on the back of my goddamned tongue itself. THE WORST F***ING CANKER SORES OF MY FREAKING LIFE. It also felt like the entire inside of my mouth was sunburned and swollen. With all of the sores and blood in my mouth, I developed breath like you wouldn't believe. Geoff started calling it "corpse breath" because it smelled like my whole mouth was rotting, which I think it effectively was.

On the positive (?) side, I lost 35 pounds more easily than any diet I have ever been on. Because the pain was so great, I really wasn't hungry, which is what made it so easy. Prior to my cancer, I had spent some significant time asking The Universe to help me drop the 25 pounds I had gained since college. Unfortunately, I was apparently not specific enough with The Universe because I didn't say, "I specifically don't want to get cancer in order to lose the weight." But I did lose the weight—and then some.

It was not that I was too tired from chemo to cook or that our fridge wasn't stocked-to-bursting from all of the food deliveries made by friends whose love language is food. My friend Kara delivered hearty bone broth (as well as other delicacies) to me as a break from chicken broth with truffle salt. My friend Kat baked loaves of mac 'n cheese that I could freeze and heat up as needed. My friend Nancy spoiled me with dishes from her local gourmet shop. My friend Paul (who owns an ice cream company) Fed-Exed buckets of ice cream in dry ice. And on and on. Friends who knew my love of food overindulged me in the most kind and thoughtful of ways, and I was so humbled and grateful for those gifts.

But I could not eat most foods because little particles of the food would find their way into my mouth sores and get stuck and rub the sores. Anything mildly astringent would sting the sores. Most days I defaulted to truffle salt chicken broth or miso soup with soft tofu if we were going out. My entire catalog of solid-ish foods was limited to poached eggs, scrambled eggs, and cottage cheese. I found when I really needed to eat, I could use a spoon to throw the food to the back of my throat thus avoiding my swollen mouth (though often hitting the sores at the back of my throat) and getting the food in me. I remember trying to eat a spoonful of cottage cheese during one of the worst weeks. Geoff was standing over me saying, "I don't think you've eaten for a couple of days. You *have* to eat something. Anything." As someone who has struggled with her weight for her entire life, this was a pretty bizarre conversation to be having. I said, "You know, sweetheart, when I gain all of this weight back, I want you to remember this day when you begged me to eat." ☺

The *really* perverse thing about all this weight loss is that folks kept telling me how great I looked. I mean, how weird is it that when I was my most sick, people thought I looked my best? And I was told that apparently beyond my shrinking size, my skin had a "glow" as well. At first, I thought these people commenting on my weight and skin were just searching around for nice things to say to me while actively avoiding discussing how *bald* I was becoming. But then I asked my dermatologist about this "glow" people kept commenting on. She explained that in the course of chemotherapy killing cancer cells, it actually kills many facial cells. The result of which was like a whole series of chemical peels/microdermabrasion to my face! Okay, so I'm going to put that in the very limited "pro" column when I finally sit down to map out the pros and cons of cancer treatment.

On the last day of radiation, I met with Dr. RadOnc so she could see the state of my mouth. I needed to hear from her that she believed my sores would now begin to heal. I figured if I was at the worst it could be, I could get through it. Unfortunately, this is when she informed me that radiation symptoms get worse for at least two weeks after the last radiation session. Ugh. So I had at least two more weeks of possibly even greater pain. I freaked myself out by reading about people who had had radiation to their mouths/esophagus and ended up in the hospital with feeding tubes and IVs full of antibiotics. I *really* didn't want that to be me.

Which brings me back to Indian Springs. We had reserved our spa day for *ten days* from my last radiation session. This had been based upon my totally uninformed belief that my mouth would be on the mend by then. Geoff asked if I wanted to postpone our spa day, but given that I had *so* been looking forward to the day away, I stubbornly said no. I wanted a day like we had had at Ventana two months earlier before I started all of these treatments.

I packed my Vera Bradley day bag with a bikini (an upside of my mouth-sore-induced weight loss), a couple of cute outfits, some magazines, and a to-go bag of mouthwashes, numbing gels, and pain meds for the day. We drove up the hour to Calistoga listening to music because my mouth sores made it too painful to speak. We checked in at the spa and were each given a day locker for our things. I met Geoff outside where he had claimed two prime real estate poolside lounge chairs. As we settled into our seats, I remembered that I was supposed to stay out of the sun as chemo can lead to greater sensitivity to the sun. We repositioned ourselves in a less desirable lounge chair neighborhood under a canopy. I tried to read my magazines but pain in my mouth grabbed all of my available attention and would not allow me to distract myself. I checked the time, decided enough time had elapsed since my last pain meds, and excused myself to go find my to-go bag.

The pain meds didn't touch the pain. In truth, the pain meds hadn't touched the pain for some time. Here's what I didn't know about prescription pain medications prior to needing them: painkillers aren't meant to *remove* the pain, but only relieve/dull it. *What*!? I wanted full removal of pain like when I would have a headache and popping an Advil removes the pain. Nope. The goal of the prescription pain meds is to relieve moderate-to-severe pain that would be felt on an extended basis (weeks/months/years) but it does not completely remove it. *Ugh.*

The doctors had tried all different kinds of meds for me. I learned that doctors categorize three levels of pain: mild-to-moderate, moderate-to-severe, and breakthrough pain. Mild-to-moderate is your daily aches and pains, like headaches or muscle soreness. This is where over-the-counter pain relievers like aspirin, Advil, and Aleve play well. Moderate-to-severe pain is treated with narcotic pain relievers like codeine, hydrocodone, or oxycodone. These are the opioids which require a prescription because they can be highly addictive.

Initially I told my breast oncologist that I didn't want opioid pain meds because I didn't want to unwittingly become addicted. She counseled that we should get through the cancer treatment however we could, and *if* I became addicted, then we'd deal with that then. And frankly, once the pain really started, I needed those meds to get through the weeks and months of pain while my body healed.

But at some point the opioids weren't working for me and I began to experience the dreaded third level of pain: "breakthrough pain." Once I had breakthrough pain, they prescribed morphine to me—which completely freaked me out as I seemed to be hurtling down the path of increasingly scary drugs. And I did not love this drug one bit. The first time I took it, I was standing in my bathroom...and the next thing I knew I was throwing up. I got no warning whatsoever about the fact that I was about to throw up because it came on so fast. One minute I was leaning toward my mirror to draw eyebrows on my face, and the next minute I was barfing onto the mirror and the counter. Oh my *God*, the indignities of this disease. I was so disgusted by this side effect of the morphine (and it didn't seem to touch the pain any better than the opioids) that I asked them to put me back on the opioids.

So on this particular day at Indian Springs, I sneaked away to the locker room to discreetly pop an opioid pill that I knew would not dull the roar of the pain in my mouth. In my head. In my body. I took a swig of my mouthwash so my breath didn't smell like a corpse. I stuck fingerful after fingerful of numbing gel into my mouth to try to relieve the topical pain of the mouth sores. I caught a glance of myself in the mirror and I saw a woman hunched over her bag of meds with thinning hair and a thinning body. I hunched more. I was the embodiment of pain. It was all I could think about. It was all I could feel. I couldn't get away from it; I couldn't get relief. I was sitting in this gorgeous resort with my thoughtful, patient husband and a luxurious day of pampering ahead of me, and all I wanted to do was go home and have a good cry.

I ducked into one of the steam rooms. Thankfully, it was empty. I sat on the wet tiles and pulled my knees up to my chest. I wrapped my arms around my knees and I buried my face in this tight little knot my body had become. I opened myself up to all of the self-pity I had been pushing away, pushing down. I rocked back and forth and I wailed. This, of course, made my mouth and throat hurt even more but somehow at this point I was beyond pain. I was just *beyond*. I rocked and I cried until I thought I had it out of me. Slowly, I stopped rocking—and eventually stopped crying—and I lay down. I let the steam surround me and hold me down. Tears mixed with sweat as I breathed in and out. "May I be well. May I be happy. May I be at peace."

.

CHAPTER TWELVE

THE F**KING GOITER (TFG)

CARINGBRIDGE ENTRY: June 13, 2012

I *LOVE* TOAST.

Mouth update. So I love toast, but unfortunately, I still can't eat it. The same crusty crispiness that I like to slather with salted butter and lemon-ginger marmalade is just too painful with my current mouth situation. And this is why you haven't received a report from me on the crunchy salad I have just eaten because sadly, I haven't eaten it as the dreaded mouth sores are still here.

*RADIATION RECALL. I've been working with the doctors on the whole-get-rid-of-these-mouth sores thing, but after a month – and a course of antibiotics, two cultures, and an injectable medicine that was supposed to boost my white blood cells – the mouth sores persist. So the doctors have decided to give me a pass on chemo this week **and next** to see if without chemo, the mouth heals. Apparently what I am experiencing with my mouth is an effect called "radiation recall." The best I can understand is that every time I have chemo, it reminds my mouth of the radiation it endured and then "recalls" it and gives the pain to me again. Bastard.*

"TFG". Part of the radiation recall effect is a lovely swelling that occurs just under my left jaw that I have affectionately begun referring to as "the f**king goiter," or "TFG" for short. I asked the doctors about "TFG" and they told me that the left side of my lymphatic system has been damaged by the radiation and is struggling to get back to working order. A working lymphatic system naturally runs fluid through it no problem, whereas mine (when I eat – or when I wake from sleeping) has trouble draining like it normally would and I end up with "TFG." And yes, the doctors are using the acronym with me now -- which I love.

Running and lifting. Other than mouth sores and TFG, I am doing just great. I have had no fatigue, no swelling, no neuropathy, no further loss of hair, blah blah blah associated with treatments. I have started running and lifting again – and even played 18 holes of golf – twice – in the last two weeks. I'm feeling dandy and am enjoying exercising. I am assured the more active I am, the better treatments go – so I am fully bought into that.

Wait. If you're on leave, can you take a vacation? Hell yes. You may have noticed that I mentioned I am not doing chemo this week – or next. Because next week the greater Brubacher family is going to Hawaii for the week! Whoo hoo! I think Hawaii is a magical place, so I am looking forward to healing there. That, and the mai-tais.

Summary metrics. Wow – the obsession with these continues. Some of the more exacting of you have pointed out to me that part of my treatment(s) has been surgery – first to the mouth and later for the breast – and that I failed to include that in my metrics. I corrected that, below. I have also added the breast radiation metrics – which had been

*a miss as well. Unfortunately, if I am inclusive of all treat-
ments, the total treatment time becomes really long...*sigh*
but that's probably appropriate for this timeline. Bottom
line, everything should be completed by about Thanksgiving.
So...here's the latest:*

Surgery. *2 total sessions/
1 completed →*   *50% complete! (new metric!)*

Mouth Radiation: *30 total
sessions/30 completed →*   *100% complete!*

Chemo I: *12 total sessions/
7 completed →*   *58% complete*

Chemo II: *4 total sessions/
0 completed →*   *0% complete (adjusted metric)*

Breast Radiation: *33 total
sessions/0 completed →*   *0% complete (new metric!)*

Total treatment: *42 total
weeks/19 completed →*   *45% complete (adjusted metric)*

Thanks for all of your love and support. Xoxo Sarah & Geoff

*   *   *

CARINGBRIDGE ENTRY: June 28, 2012

PROGRESS.

I can eat toast! *While the dang sore on the back of my tongue
is still there, I can work around it and have now successfully
eaten toast, salad, and a Tartine croissant since my last posting,
among other things. I have also been spending this week eating
as much foie gras as I can, as California has outlawed this
delicacy and the ban goes into effect July 1st, but I don't count*

the foie because it is not a pokey food. It is soft and delectable, and yes, I know I'm going to hell for loving it.

Hawaii is a magical place. The West Coast contingency of the Brubacher clan just returned from a week-long cruise among the Hawaiian Islands. My parents are big fans of cruises and have had great experiences cruising to Alaska as well as to Panama -- so Dad suggested one in Hawaii. We started in Honolulu, Oahu – sailed to Maui – then the Big Island – then Kaua'i. I have heard it quoted that 2/3 of the American populace is obese – and apparently, they all take cruises. Wow. We quickly discovered that it was easier to eat at the restaurants on board where you could be served meals rather than brave the buffet where a normal body weight is a clear competitive disadvantage. Did I mention "wow?" But the time with family was wonderful – and the time spent on the islands was delightful -- and reminded us how much we love Hawaii. I am already in the process of planning Geoff's and my next non-cruise trip to Hawaii...

Eeesh -- further loss of hair. Quite unexpectedly, my hair started falling out again while we were on the cruise. I am now at half of what was half of my hair. My sister (as sisters are meant to do) gently suggested that when we returned from the cruise I should begin scheduling my shaving party... but I'm going to see how far I can push this. During the day, I am becoming very acquainted with the hats in my wardrobe – but have become shockingly comfortable going to (nice) dinners with my patchy head uncovered.

Summary metrics. The big news this week is that I passed the 2/3 mark in chemo #I !!! Whoo hoo!!! I only have four more sessions until I am done with Taxol. Then I move on to the big guns of chemo for the months of August and

September. I have also just passed what I think is the halfway mark for total treatment. Of course, this metric can always change if treatment gets pushed out, but I am hopeful that it does not. More than 42 weeks of treatments when there are only 52 weeks in a year seems downright excessive to me, so I'm hoping to hold strong at 42 weeks.

Surgery: *2 total sessions/ 1 completed →* *Still 50% complete!*

Mouth Radiation: *30 total sessions/30 completed →* *100% complete! (completed May 8th)*

Chemo I: *12 total sessions/8 completed →* *67% complete*

Chemo II: *4 total sessions/ 0 completed →* *0% complete (scheduled to begin July 30th)*

Breast Radiation: *33 total sessions/0 completed →* *0% complete (targeted to begin in October)*

Total treatment: *42 total weeks/21 completed →* *50% complete*

Thanks for all of your love and support. Xoxo Sarah & Geoff

*   *   *

WARNING: This is a chapter where I complain a lot about the side effects I experienced. (And you thought/hoped that part of the book was over...)

Let's start with this one:

RADIATION RECALL

When I look back at the 2012 calendar, I estimate that I had mouth sores for about four months. And I gotta tell you that *four months is a really long time.* There is this weird thing about long-term pain that I didn't really understand until I had four months of pain. It is this: When you have acute pain day after day, you start to believe that it will always be this way. That you will live in this pain purgatory for the rest of your days. You will never know anything *but* pain.

I like to think of myself as a reasonably patient person, but it is tough to remain polite and upbeat to the people around you (doctors, husbands, etc.) when all you want to do is scream from the relentlessness of the pain. There was this very young, sweet resident in the breast oncology department who met with me for several of my almost-daily appointments whose name I don't even remember (so no need to shield his identity with initials). Let's instead call him SYR for "Sweet Young Resident." His first few meetings with me were great. SYR was fascinated by my medical case ("Whoa, two cancers in someone so young!?") and very eager to discuss my physical reactions to the treatments. Each meeting SYR would ask what my pain was on a scale of 1-10. I think when we started our relationship I was at a conservative 4 and it steadily climbed over the course of our meetings. First, SYR told me the pain meds they had prescribed to me *should* be reducing the pain. At our next appointment, he assured me my sores *should* be getting better. Next he told me he *could* increase the dosage if I needed, but he didn't think I should need it. When my pain had reached a level of 8, I asked if he could assess whether perhaps the sores at the back of my tongue had somehow gotten infected because they weren't getting better *and* the pain was getting worse. By about interaction number five (and pain level 9), I could no longer be polite to him. I was in excruciating pain and I needed the SYR to make it better or bring in my fully-licensed oncologist. If the meds were *dulling* my pain, I cannot even begin to imagine what that pain would have been like had I not had access to the meds. What is "manageable" pain, anyway? Pain is pain.

THE F***ING GOITER (TFG)

As if the worst f**king mouth sores of my life weren't enough, I also developed an oblong swelling under my left jaw that would appear in the mornings as I woke—and after each meal which I referred to as "the fucking goiter," or TFG for short. The doctors told me that it was my lymphatic system trying to reroute itself after the removal of my major salivary gland. It ached and swelled to the size of a large marble when it was fully inflamed. With the area under my jaw red and scorched from the radiation—and now swollen from my dysfunctional lymphatic system—I just looked weird.

I asked the SYR in breast oncology whether there was anything I could do about TFG to help the lymphatic system reroute faster. He suggested I massage the area to help move the lymphatic fluids through the system. I became obsessed with massaging it after every meal.

At my next head and neck meeting, I asked the surgeon Dr. HeadNeck about massaging TFG to reduce its size and speed the lymphatic system healing as I had been instructed by the SYR. He just shook his head. "Nope. That's just going to bruise it. Leave it alone."

I was assigned a new resident to work with.

BRUBACHER TRIP TO HAWAII

Sometime in February, Dad had started talking up the idea of a family trip to Hawaii. Now, I am actually all for *annual* trips to Hawaii and had lobbied to have this written into Geoff's and my marriage contract, but Dad's vision was that we would take a *family cruise* to the Hawaiian Islands. As in the big-white-boat-with-five-thousand-of-your-closest-friends-jammed-into-rooms-the-size-of-my-walk-in-closet kind of cruise to Hawaii.

The reason Dad was so gung-ho for this idea was multifold. For one, Dad and Mom had taken a couple of riverboat cruises in Europe and had loved them. (I suspect the fact those cruises had hundreds of people on them versus thousands may have played a role, but what do I know...) Dad loved that you could unpack once and the rest of the logistics were taken care of. He loved the concept of all-you-can-eat buffets at any time of the day or night. And in this specific case, he loved the idea that he'd be able to see four of the Hawaiian Islands over a seven-day period.

The problem was that I am married to a sailor. I have observed Geoff McDonald for over ten years now, and I honestly think he is happier when he is on water than when he is on land. He finds his footing on a sailboat. His shoulders relax. He is kinder and more empathetic because he is simply happier. But his idea of a cruise to Hawaii is racing a sailboat with a handful of friends in the Pacific Cup race from San Francisco to Hawaii. He's sailed in this race twice and it is one of those experiences that when he describes it to people, he gets a faraway look and I know he's gone to his happy place. I personally can think of few things that would terrify me more than being out on the ocean with no land in my sight, but for Geoff it is some kind of paradise.

When I got off the phone with my very enthusiastic father and shared his vision of our family vacation, I was met with:

"No, I'm not going."

"Um. Yes, you are. This is not optional."

"Oh God, Sarah, it sounds awful. I can't believe your Dad thinks this is a good idea. I really don't want to go."

I felt my heels digging in. "Geoff, this is my father's last trip. He won't be able to travel after this. It is, for all intents and purposes, his dying wish. You can't *not* go."

Pause. Pause. "Okay, but we're getting a room with a balcony."

So we did. We upgraded our room to one with a balcony. It meant we wouldn't be on the same floor with my sister and brother and their families, but given we were the only ones without young children, we figured this might actually be a good thing.

The closer we got to the actual trip, the more Dad's health deteriorated. He was relying heavily on a walker, even at home, and by the month leading up to the trip, he was occasionally using a wheelchair. I called the cruise line and upgraded Mom and Dad's room to a handicap-enabled cabin so they would have more space. I also called the airline and used all of Geoff's and my airline miles to upgrade Dad to first class.

Geoff and I flew from San Francisco while everyone else flew together from Los Angeles. We met up at the port in Honolulu and received leis for our travel efforts. Dad was visibly shaken from the long flight. It is super challenging to feel lousy over an extended period of time (see my prior screed about pain), and it's even worse when you feel lousy far from your home. Exhausted, Dad sat slumped in his wheelchair and didn't really get out of it again during the trip.

The cruise started in Oahu then sailed to Maui, the Big Island, and Kauai before returning to Oahu. At the beginning of the trip, we agreed as a group that we would individually choose how to spend our days, but would gather at the end of the day for a family dinner on the boat. Each day the ship would dock in a port and we would disembark in different pairings to explore the islands.

What Geoff and I quickly discovered is that families with small children and retired people in their seventies all sit down to eat at 5:30 pm. Geoff and I do not. We might be ready for cocktails at 5:30, but we would normally not have dinner until 7:30 or 8:00 pm. The rest of our crew liked to eat early, have baths/showers, and head to bed at 8:00 pm at the latest. 8:00 pm! Or if they weren't in bed with the kids, the adults would settle down in the hallways across from their rooms and read until they were ready for sleep. This was not our idea of how we wanted to spend a precious week of vacation.

Geoff and I decided our compromise would be to have cocktails and appetizers with the family at 5:30, and when they were all headed off for their nighttime routine, we would have dinner just the two of us. We found a sushi bar on the ship that served reasonable sushi and that became our evening routine. It was also a great way to find "us time" in the middle of a family vacation.

On Maui, Geoff and I suggested we drive Dad on the Road to Hana as he had heard it was a beautiful drive. Geoff and I awkwardly got Dad from his wheelchair into the front seat and then optimistically drove off. The Road to Hana is lush and green with little excursions to waterfalls and other scenic views that you can pull off to see. But it is also 64 miles of hairpin turns, and it turns out Dad doesn't like winding roads. And because he was unsteady on his feet, getting out to explore waterfalls along the way to break up the drive wasn't going to work. So after several miles of Dad telling us he might throw up, we double-backed and decided to play to our strengths—eating. Following our maps, we made our way to Mama's Fish House for lunch. Mama's is absurdly overpriced, but the view was stunning and getting food in Dad's stomach was critical.

It was hard to be with Dad on this trip. I know that is a terrible thing to say; I know. You would think or hope that when you know your time with someone is short, each moment together is poignant and heartbreakingly memorable. But the reality can be different. It was/is complicated to spend time with someone who is dying. Who knows he is dying. Dad felt lousy every minute of every day. He still had the hangover of the prior week's chemo, leaving him parched, headachy, and nauseated during his waking hours. His movement was limited by legs he could no longer trust to hold him up, and he was increasingly confined to a wheelchair on a ship where he couldn't trust the listing of the deck any more than he could trust his legs. He was suffering the indignity of adult diapers, the discomfort of that non-breathable, padded material, the constant scent of urine, the inconvenience of needing an extra set in the event the current diaper became heavy and unwearable. And those were just the physical reminders of his cancer. Even harder for him—and for all of us—was the unspoken knowledge we all had that this was our last trip together. Dad's physical challenges were no longer ones he would bounce back from. The path forward was becoming increasingly clear, and the timeline felt like it was accelerating.

This whole family trip was hard. All of the physical abuses Dad was experiencing made him cranky. He could no longer bear his physical insults alone. He willingly overshared his physical indignities. He was quick to anger and frustratingly critical of all of us. My joking, thoughtful father was a distant memory. In his place was a very tired curmudgeon just trying to get through each day. The rest of us responded by overplaying the *fun* we were having on the trip. At dinner we recounted the stories from our days on the islands to one another, each story of play with one another more camp-y than the last. We told Dad we were having an *amazing, hilarious* trip together and avoided discussing what was too hard to say out loud.

We had two days on Kauai. Day One we sent Mom and Dad on a helicopter ride over the island—a first for both of them—while the rest of us took a break from my cranky father and enjoyed Poipu Beach for the day. Day Two, Geoff and I drove Mom and Dad up to Hanalei to have lunch at the St. Regis in Princeville where we had spent our honeymoon. The main restaurant looks out over Hanalei Bay where (if you squint) the mountains look like a dragon and inspired the song "Puff, the Magic Dragon." Afterward, we drove up the Kuhio Highway to the jumping-off spot for hiking the Na Pali Coast. This part of Kauai was full of memories for Geoff and me. We wanted Mom and Dad to experience those places the way we had—to have some of the love we felt when returning rub off on them and make them happy.

Vacation is meant to be a time to get away from the day-to-day realities of your life, but with cancer, there was no getting away from it. Cancer wasn't invited on this vacation, but it stubbornly reminded us of its presence with Dad's wheelchair, his diapers, and his fatigue. Dad sat sullenly at lunch and refused to get out of the car when we stopped to look at the water on the Kuhio Highway. I wanted to distract my father—help him turn off the Cancer Channel if only for a day—but it felt like the cancer voice in his head was louder than anything I could drown out.

I spent a lot of time on that trip sitting on our balcony watching the water go by. I tried to tell myself that what was happening to Dad wasn't necessarily what would happen to me. I tried to tell myself that we had different cancers, or that perhaps all of my treatments would be more effective than his had been, or that the fact I was being so aggressive with my treatments would save me, or that I was younger. But it was hard to watch my father's decline and not wonder when mine would begin. I tried to focus on the present moment and breathe through my fear. I took mental snapshots of the islands that I could replay for myself during acupuncture sessions. I asked the magical Hawaiian Islands to help heal me. I asked the islands to bring my Dad some relief, a respite from his physical, mental, and emotional pain. I asked cancer to be gentle with him as it slowly took his life.

LOSS OF TASTE

In August, after the mouth sores were mostly gone and I could start eating again, I lost my sense of taste. It was an added insult to injury.

All food took on a kind of bland quality, like I had cotton wrapped around my tongue. I counteracted it by seeking out more flavor. Pizza with a red sauce (and really, *any* Italian food) became my go-to. And if I hadn't been a liberal user of salt previously (actually, I had), it became a critical ingredient for me if I hoped to detect any flavor. I did not understand how much my taste had been impacted until one night when I was cooking a big batch of split pea soup. Geoff brought home a deep dish pizza from our favorite local pizzeria, Little Star Pizza. I was putting the finishing touches on the split pea soup by adding salt and pepper for taste as Geoff served up slices of the pizza. Ignoring his protests that it would be too much food, I ladled out a cup of split pea soup, the masterpiece I had just created, for Geoff to taste.

I sat down and took a large bite of the pizza and almost immediately spit it back out. "Oh God," I said. "What did they *do* to this pizza tonight? It is awful."

"Tastes the same to me," Geoff told me. "In fact, I think it is particularly good tonight."

Horror-stricken, I told him, "Do not taste the soup…"

CHAPTER THIRTEEN

TEAM TWO

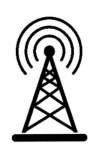

CARINGBRIDGE ENTRY: July 23, 2012

CHEMO 1 COMPLETE!

*Chemo 1 milestone achieved. WHOO HOO! Today I finished
my last infusion of "taxol." As I believe I've mentioned
in other posts – I have been super lucky with this chemo
protocol and have experienced very few side effects. Other
than the chemo slowing the mouth recovery – and the hair
loss (which wasn't even all of my hair!) – this has been a
pretty gentle experience. Yay. I needed that.*

*Chemo 2 starts Monday, July 30th → Bring it on. We
discussed with the doctor and decided there was no reason
to take a break between chemo protocols given how well
my body was responding to the taxol (tumor is shrinking,
lymph nodes can no longer be "palpated"). MONDAY I start
the next chemo medicine whose names are Adriamycin and
Cytoxan – also known as "A/C." This medicine will be given to
me every other week – so I'll have a week on and a week off.
I will do four infusions for a total of eight weeks. So far, we
have planned that on the first "off" week I will travel to visit*

Geoff's family in Connecticut – and for the 2nd "off" week, my family in Southern California. There is the possibility that my immune system will be suppressed so I will travel with antibiotics - but truly, we do not expect any issues.

Did someone say HEADSHAVE? Just a reminder if you missed that last post that the Head Shaving Party is scheduled for 7pm Wednesday, August 1st. We will toast to baldness and then we will turn the clipper on this patchy head.

Summary metrics. HA! I have two major metrics that stand at 100%!!

Surgery: 2 total sessions/ 1 completed → Still 50% complete! (Surgery 2 targeted for early October)

Mouth Radiation: 30 total sessions/30 completed → 100% complete! (completed May 8th)

Chemo I: 12 total sessions/ 12 completed → 100% complete! (completed July 23rd)

Chemo II: 4 total sessions/ 0 completed → 0% complete (scheduled to begin July 30th)

Breast Radiation: 33 total sessions/0 completed → 0% complete (targeted to begin in November)

Total treatment: 42 total weeks/25 completed → 60% complete

Thanks for all of your love and support. Xoxo Sarah & Geoff

*   *   *

CARINGBRIDGE ENTRY: August 7, 2012

BALD IS BEAUTIFUL.

*I am **BALD**. After much ado, we **finally** had the head shaving party on August 1st. By my count, I have now had one week of baldness and so far, it is GREAT. It is MUCH better than that patchy, thin, aging hair I was sporting before. (Someone who doesn't know my mother actually mistook me for my mother. MY GOD – time to shave!) The party was a success -- my head was shaved, everyone sipped champagne, and there were pictures taken. I promise I will upload the evidence as soon as I figure out how to do it...*

*__CLEAN MRI.__ This is the single best news we have received since my initial diagnosis in January. Last week I had a head and neck MRI to see if there was any trace of cancer left in my head or neck region (either a recurrence at the site of the tumor – or cancer that might have – gulp – metastasized). As you can imagine, this is a nerve-wracking experience... especially waiting for the results. But the results came up totally clean – with "no definite findings of perineural invasion." Translated: this wonderful, glorious MRI shows no evidence of cancer at the site of the tumor, in the brain, in the lungs, or in those pesky nerves. **This is tremendous news!!***

Background: You'll remember that when the doctor excised the tumor, he felt he had gotten clean margins (removed the tumor intact – with no cancer cells present for a centimeter around it). In the labs, the tech suggested that some cancer cells may have been making footsteps toward my nerve with the goal of heading to my brain...So we made the aggressive decision to do radiation to blow any possible cancer cells out of the region...and blow we did. HA! Take that, mofo cancer! This clean MRI makes all of those painful mouth sores totally worth it, I can tell you.

CHEMO 2 has begun. I had my first badass chemo infusion on July 30th and it wasn't bad. The side effects were kind of like having a mild hangover that you can't shake. I had a headache, was slightly nauseated, and wasn't interested in eating. Luckily, my life before cancer had prepared me well to know how to deal with a hangover, so I was a-okay... That – and some good friends of ours who live in Belvedere on the lagoon were on vacation for the week of my infusion and offered us their home for my recovery...So recover I did – lying on a deck chair in view of the sun-speckled waters – Marin breezes lightly caressing me – book in hand and ice water and Advil at the ready. Easy peasy. Bring it on, Chemo 2 – I know how to deal with you.

Summary metrics. I only have four sessions of chemo 2 (every other week), so I am already 25% of the way through. I LOVE metrics like that.

Surgery: 2 total sessions/1 completed	Still 50% complete
Mouth Radiation: 30 total sessions/30 completed	100% complete! (completed May 8th)
Chemo I: 12 total sessions/12 completed	100% complete! (completed July 23rd)
Chemo II: 4 total sessions/1 completed	25% complete!!!!! YAY!!!!!
Breast Radiation: 33 total sessions/0 completed	0% complete
Total treatment: 42 total weeks/27 completed	64% complete (Go faster, you dumb metric.)

Thanks for all of your love and support. Xoxo Sarah & Geoff

*   *   *

SUSAN'S MOTHER

It wasn't until I went to see a performance my sister Susan was in and a friend of hers stopped me to ask, "Are you Susan's mother?" that I thought I really needed to deal with the thinning hair situation and shave my head. So I did. About a dozen friends showed up and each was invited to shave a portion of my hair off.

Sitting in front of a wall of mirrors, we shaved my head down to a mohawk and then completely clean. Geoff documented the whole thing with photos and then I took selfies with each person at the party. I laughed to the point of crying and realized crying is really what I wanted to do. After the shaving party, Geoff and I had dinner in that neighborhood with our friends Katherine and Rick. I had brought a really colorful red, orange, and white scarf that I tied around my head. The scarf looked great with my outfit, but it felt like I had now assumed the guise of the cancer patient. I did my best not to think about it, but it was hard. And bald went on for days, then weeks, then months.

I was bald from August until about December. Some days I was totally fine with it and would even go grocery shopping without a scarf or hat or wig (though this was really pretty cold in San Francisco!). Walking through Trader Joe's shopping with a completely bald head tricked me into believing that I had accepted my baldness and was very brave. But not every day was like that.

CULINARY GIRLS WEEKEND

During my time at Le Cordon Bleu culinary school, I met two of my best girlfriends, Amy and Lea. When I moved to San Francisco in 2003, Amy and Lea announced they wanted to help me celebrate my birthday. We chose the last weekend in October for our get together in my new hometown. As it was Halloween, I picked them up at the airport in a

Thing One costume with shocking blue hair/white face/red union suit and whisked them away to a party in the Castro. This inaugurated what has become our annual culinary girls' weekend. Each year we choose a different west coast city to explore. We focus on cooking and eating and wine tasting, but most importantly, laughing and sharing the stories of our lives with one another.

Amy and Lea checked in to see if I was up for our annual trip. Um, hell yes.

I suggested the last weekend in September hoping enough time would have passed from my last chemo infusion that I would have my sense of taste back. It was my first night away from Geoff or my family since being diagnosed, and I was excited to do something completely on my own and not cancer-related. It felt like cancer had been going on *for so long*—nine whole months! I wanted to feel like it was normal for me to go away for a weekend. Like I had time to waste. Like I didn't have cancer.

We chose Portland, Oregon (Amy lives there) and met up Friday night at a restaurant called Pok-Pok that has truly superb Thai food. Amy did all of the ordering. The three of us hadn't seen one another since the whole cancer mayhem had started, so our first night together was spent sharing the big life events of the past year. Obviously, I had many stories to choose from, but it was hard to know how to sum up all of the medical and emotional experiences I had been through (and was still going through). I decided to give them the highlight reel and then tried to be as light and funny as I could be to make all of us feel more comfortable with the subject of my cancer. They followed suit with their stories and we were all quickly laughing and diving into the food delivered to our table.

I was really hungry and took a healthy portion of each dish Amy had selected. As I shoveled the delicious food into my mouth, I began to notice how (wow!) spicy it was. And the more I put into my mouth, the more I noticed TFG starting to swell just below the left side of my jaw. I drank ice water to try to cool the area. I tried to surreptitiously massage it so the swelling would go down. All the while I was watching Amy and Lea talking and willing them not to notice my distress. Suddenly Amy stopped mid-sentence and looked directly at me with shocked concern. "Are you okay?"

My mouth felt sunburned like it had when I was going through radiation. TFG was super painful and I didn't seem to be able to do anything to calm it down. Amy offered to order some other less spicy dishes but I told her not to. I was embarrassed and defeated and just wanted the meal to be over. Here I was with two of my closest girlfriends, and all I wanted to do was be by myself so that I could have a big ugly cry and feel sorry for myself. I wanted so desperately to have a *normal* weekend and here was my cancer reminding me how very far from normal I still was.

We spent Saturday wine tasting in the Willamette Valley at various wineries Amy represented. As my palate was just starting to recognize wine as something more palatable than lighter fluid, I was conservative in my tasting, but still participated at every winery. Lea (nickname: Captain Picnic) planned a picnic and had brought with her some favorite recent food discoveries for us to sample (think salami, cheese, foie gras in a jar). Amy supplemented the meal with bread and butter pickles she had made and fruits she had canned, all from her own garden. These women are the real deal. I sat on a picnic bench in the late September sunshine, grateful for the bounty both of food and of dear friends.

For fun, I had brought all of my (now three!) wigs with me so that Lea and Amy could each choose to wear one to our big dinner Saturday night if they wanted. Which of course they did. Amy chose the short red wig and Lea chose the blonde wig. They both looked fabulous and had the *best* time changing their look for the evening, taking photos to send to their husbands. I really did think they both looked gorgeous, but I couldn't help thinking that at the end of the evening they could take the wigs off and go back to their beautiful hair while I was still bald. And once that got into my head, I spent our big night out feeling sorry for myself, again. I tried to keep up with all of the laughter, but what I really wanted to do was go back to the hotel and have a good cry.

In the hotel, Amy and Lea gave me my own bed and they shared the other queen. I think instinctively they knew I needed some space both physically and emotionally that weekend. We talked non-stop because that is what the three of us do. They both asked questions about cancer, but mostly what they did was assure me that everything would get back to normal—that our culinary girls' weekends would continue and we (read: I) would be alright.

ACUPUNCTURE

As captain of Team Two, Tripti suggested that beyond the yoga, meditation, and energy work I was doing, I should also pursue acupuncture. I had tried acupuncture when I was going through fertility treatments. Frankly, while I thought Amanda, the fertility acupuncturist, was delightful, I found the acupuncture itself uncomfortable and oftentimes painful. Other girlfriends of mine who were focused on getting pregnant told me they loved it—it was the guaranteed hour-long nap they looked forward to each week. In contrast, I found myself wide awake and staring at the ceiling—and breathing through the discomfort of the needles.

When I was first receiving acupuncture treatment for my fertility issues, Amanda focused on inserting needles along the left side of my body. Apparently the meridian that goes up the left side of the body is the one that controls fertility. When Amanda was inserting needles, my body felt like it was being sunburned. The needles stung and I couldn't get comfortable.

When Tripti suggested I try acupuncture again, she sent me to a dear friend of hers in Half Moon Bay named Lisa. Tripti assured me that

Lisa worked with cancer patients regularly and knew the side effects of treatments and how to relieve them. I thought to myself, *Well, it can't hurt—and it might help*, and made my way to her office.

Lisa would start each session sitting across from me, taking my wrists in each hand, and feeling for my pulse. She would then ask to see my tongue and would ask how my bowel movements were. At first I felt a little awkward about this line of questioning, but decided that if I was going to give acupuncture a real try, I needed to be real honest.

Lisa set me up in a small room with a 30-foot-high ceiling that had a large window up at the top. I could hear birds chirping happily at me while I undressed to my skivvies, covered myself with a sheet, and lay down on the therapy bed. Lisa efficiently and gently twisted needles into me and then asked if I wanted to listen to music while the needles worked. Yes, please.

Lisa placed headphones over my ears and walked away, closing the door. Gorgeous slack-key guitar notes felt like they were playing in the middle of my head and reminded me of prior trips to Hawaii. I relaxed and was surprised when Lisa returned that I had drifted off to sleep.

So began my love of acupuncture, slack key, and Lisa.

Did I have less pain due to acupuncture? Fewer hot flashes? Less constipation? Maybe. It is hard to say what worked directly on my side effects as I was trying so many different things. What I will tell you is that I was absolutely more relaxed.

Sometimes I think back to how the fertility acupuncture didn't work because I didn't get pregnant. About three months into my acupuncture relationship with Lisa, I told her how much I had disliked the fertility acupuncture. I told her of the stinging and the sunburn feeling and the discomfort. And how I wasn't experiencing that now. Acupuncture now was painless and relaxing, and something I looked forward to each week.

"You know the fertility meridian ends on the left side of the floor of your mouth, right? Just under your tongue?"

Wait. Where I had had the salivary gland tumor?

So here's the thing I noodle on every once in a while...

Is it possible that the fertility acupuncture was painful *because* I had a tumor at the end of the meridian that controls fertility? And/or was I having trouble with fertility *because* there was a tumor at the end of the meridian? And/or did stimulating the qi in that meridian send any bad stuff that got stuck at the end of the meridian to become a tumor?

CHAPTER FOURTEEN

WE MAKE THE BEST DECISIONS WE CAN

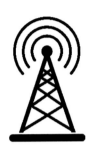

CARINGBRIDGE ENTRY: September 11, 2012

BADASS CHEMO COMPLETE!

All chemo is finished as of yesterday. *Wow, this has been a long time coming! I looked in my calendar and saw that my chemo program started March 27th – over five months ago...I am so thrilled to be on this side of that mountain – whew!*

How am I doing? *I'm doing just great. I mean – yes – the next two weeks won't be my best as the medicine works its way through my body. I'm experiencing side effects – but honestly, mine have really been pretty mild in comparison to other stories I hear. Oh, side effects – let me count the ways...Chemo dries everything out – so I am parched. I am never far from a large glass of water with ice. I have nausea – but as I've quipped – my pre-cancer life taught me how to power through a hangover. I don't have much appetite and have "radiation recall" again in my mouth – so the combination makes eating less interesting – but* it's really getting fascinating to see how much weight I can actually lose. I'm at 30 lbs lost right now – at a weight I haven't seen since high school! (Wow.) And oh yes – I am still bald – but I am already starting to scout out pixie haircuts I can sport once I have approximately two(?) inches of hair on my head. The question is whether I should dye it platinum blonde...

So, what's next? I will have an MRI the week of the 17th to see how much the tumor has shrunk – and whether the disease is still in my lymph nodes. Then I will meet with the breast surgeon to negotiate my surgery date (I will push for early October). Approximately three weeks after the breast surgery, I will begin six weeks of radiation to my left breast. Thankfully, the breast radiation is meant to be much easier than the mouth radiation I received previously. I'll probably experience fatigue and a "sunburn" associated with it – but I should still be able to eat – for which I am already grateful. And after radiation is complete...my year of cancer will be finished. Hooray.

So (cough) what surgery will I have? It is totally okay to ask that question. Hell, I've been talking with you people about my breasts since March – so I'm happy to share with you what way Geoff and I are leaning. Our current thinking is that I will have a lumpectomy rather than a double mastectomy. My reasons for choosing a lumpectomy over a mastectomy are both practical and emotional:

- Per the doctors, the survivorship metrics for both paths are comparable. 95% long-term survivorship for mastectomies and 90% long-term survivorship for lumpectomies – so 5% difference. (Note: I like these metrics *that are in the 90s! Of course I would prefer 100% – but while breast oncology has made huge leaps in the last decade – they're not at 100% yet.)*

- I will have to do radiation regardless of the path I choose. And radiation doesn't work well with "reconstruction." Initially, I had misunderstood that I could do the mastectomy and reconstruction during the same surgery – and if I did the mastectomy I could avoid another round of radiation. Sadly, I believe I was wrong on both accounts.

*- Mastectomies are **major** surgery. They take longer to recover from than a lumpectomy. You may remember that I started this journey in January (diagnosis #1) and I am hesitant to add additional weeks/months to my journey when we're already at almost a full year.*

- The most compelling benefit I could see from a double mastectomy was that I would never need to wear a strapless bra again. And – while it was (dare I use the word) titillating to contemplate my future halter dresses – it seemed a poor reason for me (personally) to undergo major surgery.

- I can always choose a mastectomy later. While doing a lumpectomy still allows you to choose a mastectomy in the future, the opposite is not true. This is the #1 reason my surgeon gave me that I should consider a lumpectomy. He says he has a lot of patients who make the emotional decision to have a mastectomy (I was certainly in that camp when first diagnosed) who then regret the decision due to the long, painful path to recovery.

***Summary metrics.** I am excited to be reporting I am at 100% for 3 of my 6 metrics now. Whoo hoo!*

Surgery: 2 total sessions/1 completed	Still 50% complete! (Breast surgery targeted for early October)
Mouth Radiation: 30 total sessions/30 completed	100% complete! (completed May 8th)
Chemo I: 12 total sessions/12 completed	100% complete! (completed July 23rd)
Chemo II: 4 total sessions/4 completed	100% complete! (completed September 10th)
Breast Radiation: 33 total sessions/0 completed	0% complete (targeted to begin in November)
Total treatment: 42 total weeks/32 completed	76% complete

Thanks for all of your love and support. Xoxo Sarah & Geoff

*   *   *

CARINGBRIDGE ENTRY: *October 22, 2012*

LONG TIME, NO POST.

Yes, I agree. It has been a crazy couple of weeks – so I haven't blogged as I probably should have. Let me bring you up to date now.

SURGERY. When last we left our heroine, she was waiting for the next step in the journey – a lumpectomy...

Third time's the charm. Prior to scheduling the surgery, the doctors asked that I have a mammogram, a sonogram, a CT scan, and an MRI to "see how things were looking" and ensure I was still a candidate for a lumpectomy. Three of the four scans went off with no hitches – but I had some challenges with the MRI. When the doctors reviewed the

MRI, they found the scan "cut off" halfway through the visual of the tumor. GAH! 45 minutes facedown in a casket-like tube listening to a deafening knocking sound and the scan didn't capture a picture of the tumor!?!? So it was back to the claustrophobia tube for me for another try...and wouldn't you know it — during the very last scan they did (injecting a contrast dye into me via an IV) – it didn't work AGAIN!?!? I got halfway home only to receive a phone call to turn around and head back down to Stanford for a third MRI. Whew – but I knew it was important to get the best pictures we could prior to the surgery.

Except that it wasn't charming. *Unfortunately, the third MRI (now clear pictures) showed another "area of enlargement" on the scan. Oh my God – WHAT is an "area of enlargement"? MRIs highlight areas of blood flow. Cancer has to find a blood source to feed it – so when you look at an MRI with a malignancy – the area will be "lit up" with blood flow (think Lite-Brite pegs). My third MRI showed a brightly lit, but much-reduced original tumor (good) and another brightly lit area that hadn't been seen in any prior MRIs (bad). With all this I'm thinking – I've just gone through FIVE MONTHS of chemotherapy and now there's some kind of new chemotherapy-resistant tumor? Based upon this breaking news, I started a one-woman campaign for an immediate double mastectomy. My surgeon (who apparently has more knowledge of this whole cancer thing than I do) — and my husband — both proved to have cooler heads than I and talked me off the ledge. My surgeon's recommendation was an MRI-guided biopsy (of COURSE another MRI!) to determine exactly what it was. No need for a mastectomy if it is just breast tissue, he reasoned with me. So — biopsy we did and they took out a full gram*

*(!!) of the area. Thus began our next waiting period —
not unlike the waiting Geoff and I had gone through with
the initial diagnosis. Now we were wondering if the good
prognoses we had been counting on had suddenly changed.
Thankfully, the pathology came back benign – and we are
reminded again how very lucky we are.*

God and the angels. *At the end of the above rollercoaster
two weeks, my father quietly lost his battle with metastatic
prostate cancer. I know. It's a lot. Thankfully, he wasn't in
any pain and died peacefully. Our whole family was able to
spend the week prior with him and we all had a chance to
tell him how much we loved him. It was as much of a blessing as we could ask for in what we knew was a totally lousy
eventuality...Recently, I listened to this great NPR article
about a comedienne's (Tig Notaro) standup routine based
upon all of the tough things that had been going on in her
life all at once – like getting diagnosed with breast cancer,
losing her mother, and ending her primary relationship. She
talked about how people always say that "God only gives you
as much as you can handle." So she envisioned God standing
around with the angels – and the angels saying, "No, God!
Don't give her anything more – it's too much!" And God looking at the angels — weighing this possibility — and saying
"Actually – I think she can take a little bit more..." Boy, Geoff
and I laughed at that as it has definitely felt like that this
year. Bring on 2013!*

Out, out, damned cancer!! *On Wednesday of last week,
I checked into Stanford Hospital at 6:00 am to begin
preparations (read: more tests) for my surgery at 2:45 pm
(6:00 am!!). The good news was that we were so efficient
with all of these tests that I was moved up on the schedule by
three hours. THREE HOURS!! I cannot begin to tell you how*

tremendous that was. The nurses at Stanford were following a strict no-water-prior-to-surgery rule with me (since 6:00 am!!). This was pure torture given the dry mouth I am still experiencing due to the salivary gland surgery. Moving my surgery up by three hours meant three hours closer to ice chips and eventually the gallons of water I was fantasizing about. Luckily, my rule-breaking brother smuggled in a small cup of water to allow me to wet the back of my aching throat - relief! Post-surgery, I spent an hour in the recovery room (sucking on ice chips) and then was released to GO HOME!! Whoo hoo! No night in the hospital for me. In celebration, I had pizza (not hospital jello) and at least a gallon of water for dinner.

I feel great. Post-surgery I'm sore and a little swollen, but basically feeling great. The surgeon told us he believes he got it all out and that it went "as well as he could have hoped for". I'll have my follow-up meetings with my surgeon and oncologist later this week to review the pathology and confirm his confidence. And in a couple of weeks I'll begin radiation to the left breast – the final part of my treatment. I am feeling very CANCER-FREE these days and that is a wonderful feeling.

Summary metrics. Yet another key metric moved to 100% complete. Surgeries for both the left salivary gland and the left breast are complete!!

Surgery: 2 total sessions/2 completed	100% complete! (February 7th & Oct 17th)
Mouth Radiation: 30 total sessions/30 completed	100% complete! (completed May 8th)
Chemo I: 12 total sessions/ 12 completed	100% complete! (completed July 23rd)

Chemo II: *4 total sessions/4 completed*	*100% complete! (completed Sept 10th)*
Breast Radiation: *33 total sessions/0 completed*	*0% complete*
Total treatment: *47 total weeks/37 completed*	*79% complete (Adjusted to reflect the new treatment timeline — estimated treatment end date of December 21st)*

Thanks for all of your love and support. Xoxo Sarah & Geoff

*   *   *

Over the course of my multi-month chemotherapy, I had become pretty comfortable with the routine of my treatments: Get up. Shower. Wear cute outfit. Drive with scheduled friend (Geoff/Bruno/Nancy/Tami etc.) to Stanford. Sit for four hours in a beige pleather La-Z Boy while drugs course through my body. Drive home. Pizza dinner. Spend the week meeting friends for lunch, working out, exploring my city. My appointments with my oncologist were very encouraging, e.g. "The lump has definitely reduced in size with the chemotherapy, Sarah" or "Wow, you're doing great, Sarah—you are responding so well to treatment." I began to have a swagger of cautious confidence that perhaps they really *could* cure me of the breast cancer.

In the two weeks leading up to my surgery, I did another battery of tests. Armed with cautious confidence, I charmed my way through each test. I joked with the technicians. I held my breath when I was told to. I twisted into each uncomfortable position for as long as the technician asked. Eventually, all of the tests were complete and it was just a matter of waiting for the results to confirm what I already knew—that the tumor was reducing and the scheduled lumpectomy was merely the next step in the eventuality of my cure.

DAD IS MY CANCER TWIN

A number of cancer book authors (Kelly Corrigan in *The Middle Place*, Nina Riggs in *The Bright Hour*) have written about what it is like to have cancer at the same time as a parent. It is sad and crushing, and it is hard not to watch the progression of disease in your parent and not wonder if it is the bellwether for your own imminent death.

Going through cancer treatments at the same time is depressing, but—I have to guiltily admit—less lonely. Dad and I would call one another almost every day, which was new for us. We had always been good for the weekly parental check-in phone calls, but now it was quick daily check-ins for both of us. We would compare doctors' appointments and bodily reactions to treatments. Neither of us was working full time while we made time for our treatments, so we regularly talked in the middle of the day and didn't risk interrupting the other from some other, more important task. What could we possibly be doing that was more important than our cancer treatments? When he couldn't reach me directly, Dad would leave singing messages for me like the one where he sang (to the tune of "Hello, Dolly") "Well, hello, Sari—yes, hello, Sari!" and then shared with me his triumph of completing a full-circuit walk around their house. This from the father whose prior triumphs included playing competitive tennis in college but who now would not have been able to walk the circumference of a tennis court without a walker.

Dad decided to start chemotherapy sometime in the summer of 2012. Since I was having so little (bad) reaction to my chemo, I regularly flew down to Southern California after *my* infusion days to be with him after *his* infusion days. Unfortunately, Dad's body didn't react as well to his chemo cocktail as mine did for what were probably a number of reasons. For one, he and I were being given different chemotherapies based upon our different cancers. Also, his cancer had spread to his bones and his liver by the time his doctors realized it had returned. And given that Dad had stopped playing tennis in his sixties, his aerobic shape had really deteriorated. Chemo left him exhausted and nauseated and ultimately, it did little to slow the progression of his disease. His weeks post-infusion were exhausting, punctuated by bouts of nausea. It was hard.

"I just don't understand how, if we have the same bodies, yours is reacting well to the chemo and mine isn't," he said to me.

"I have no answer, Dad," I said, feeling frustrated that I was getting better and he wasn't.

Our conversations were long and they were short. We could discuss insignificant issues like what our current favorite way to scramble eggs was (green onion + shredded cheddar + "soft" scramble), or weighty issues like whether chemo was worth it if you felt lousy all the time. Sometimes it just felt good to hear his voice and know he was going through what I was going through, like a touchstone with my cancer twin.

Then one Sunday in September I called home for the weekly scheduled parental check-in and Mom got on the phone at the same time with Dad. That wasn't unusual per se except that this night, Mom was the only one talking. Dad was silent. I asked Dad a couple of questions directly and he said nothing. Mom said, "He's nodding at the phone, Sarah, but he doesn't seem to be able to speak to the phone. He really seems to be having trouble talking today."

"Mom, I just spoke with him *yesterday*. What changed? We have to call his doctor immediately. There must be something they can do. Maybe he has an infection in his brain? Mom, we have to *do* something. I can fly down this week to help make it happen." I remember saying this to her, trying hard to tamp down the hysteria I was feeling. Was this the beginning of my Dad dying? Or had he been dying and I just hadn't kept up? Had I just had my last conversation with him and I didn't know it? What would I have said to him if I had known it was the last time we would ever speak?

I called both my brother and sister and we talked through what we might do to help Mom and Dad. The doctors insisted Dad would have to come to the office to be seen. (Why couldn't they make house calls to someone so clearly in distress? Didn't they understand my father was *dying*!? Where was their sense of urgency?) Doctor visits were getting increasingly difficult for my Mom as Dad was heavy to lift and in this new state, really unable to understand how he needed to help Mom get him into the car. My brother David and I flew down from San Francisco for a couple of days to help.

Of the siblings, I think David and I look the most alike—which is saying something, as Susan and I have spent the majority of our lives assuring people that we are not twins. David began shaving his head in his mid-twenties when his hairline started abandoning him, so here we were, David and me, both bald. Dad in his confused state kept referring to me as "David" when he could talk, and then giggling to himself when I would correct him that I was actually Sarah. It is my favorite memory from this time and how I love to remember him—giggling at himself.

Mom had picked up some literature from the local hospice care group which we all began to study like it was midterm exams. The booklet about the final stage prior to death warned us that he would become more and more confused as time went on. We could expect him to start looking past us when we spoke to him. We were told he would begin balling up pieces of tissue (what!?) and scattering them around. (Um, wow. He totally did this. How did the hospice people know?) It was one of the most poorly written booklets I have ever read, but it accurately outlined all of the bizarre behavior my Dad was exhibiting— all of the signs that death was near were now laid out in that poorly written prose.

It was a helpless week. Collectively, we were wholly consumed with getting Dad to the doctor to "fix" him. There was blood in his urine I wanted them to test. Did he have an infection? Could they get him on antibiotics? He had only a sporadic ability to talk, and when he did, he was confused. Did this mean the cancer was in his brain, or was this the infection? It felt like we were watching a boxing match with cancer landing body blow after body blow and my father could do little to shield himself. I was outraged that his medical team didn't seem to have the same sense of urgency we did. I felt that when I had a physical issue (like sores in my mouth), my medical team explored every option to "fix" it. Where was this level of care for my father? Then slowly, I began to wonder if his team knew something we didn't know. Maybe they weren't doing anything about the blood in his urine because they knew there was nothing left to do.

Objectively, I knew Dad was dying. I knew the time would come when his body couldn't take another blow. But emotionally, I couldn't keep up. I had always loved my father, but as my cancer twin, now I craved him. He was part of my every day. For nine months we had shared cancer—the good, the bad, and now, the ugly. He had been my cancer forerunner, and now he was dying. He was losing his match with cancer. Would this mean I would lose mine?

I had been home in southern California for five days when my surgeon's PA called me. She told me the pathology had come back from the MRI and the doctors saw an "area of enlargement" that concerned them. This is the scare I mentioned in the CaringBridge entry at the beginning of the chapter.

Cancer is a roller coaster. One day you are on the path to recovery—it's been a hard, upward climb on a rickety frame—but you feel like you're finally at the top of the hill. You can see your future, or at least some glimmer of it. The next day, a test comes back and the security of your seat falls away from you. You freefall as the doctors try to interpret the results and plot your next moves.

The PA recommended we do an MRI-guided biopsy to determine exactly what this area was. She wanted to know how quickly I could come in. I told her I was in Southern California because my father was dying from cancer. Her voice changed as she told me how sorry she was. Then she asked if I could be at Stanford in two days so they could perform the biopsy. I told her I would change my flight and see her Friday.

My siblings and I talked with Mom and gently suggested it was time for us to bring in a hospice nurse to help with Dad's care. Mom agreed it had become too hard for her to care for him physically. We contacted a hospice. I flew home.

The hospice nurse met with us the next morning and thanks to the wonders of Skype, my brother set me up on a laptop in my parents' sunroom (where Dad's hospital bed now was) so we could *all* meet with the hospice nurse. We spoke to her of our desire for Dad to be kept comfortable, and for Mom to be supported (especially physically) as she cared for him. At the end of the meeting, David carried my laptop over to Dad so I could tell him I loved him, and that I would be back down to see him the week after my surgery should all go according to plan. Dad, now well beyond words, just smiled at the laptop.

I headed to Stanford again. While I wasn't crazy about getting into a small tube again, this one had an opening to the side so they had access to my breast in order to drill into it to pull out a gram (!) of flesh to biopsy. I bruised awfully (purple, green) from this biopsy, but I didn't care. I was still freefalling on the roller coaster and just wanted to hit the bottom and know what we were dealing with.

The pathology came back benign. They didn't know why the area had lit up ("sometimes it just happens"), but the biopsy told them it was nothing. We could move forward with the lumpectomy on Wednesday. I breathed again and began riding the roller coaster back up.

No longer able to have my daily phone calls with Dad, I called Mom with my great pathology news. I also wanted to be assured that the hospice nurse had shown up to help her and that somehow, *now* everything would be okay. The nurse would get the infection I was convinced he had under control. He would feel better, he would be less confused, he would be able to talk with me again. We would resume our daily phone calls for the time he had left. Dad might not recover, but he would return to the Dad I remembered and missed.

Mom confirmed that the nurse had arrived, but she told me Dad was in and out of consciousness and his breathing had changed. He was making a rattle sound which was very jarring to listen to, but which the hospice booklet assured Mom was not painful for him. The rest of the conversation was spent discussing how to get morphine into him to ease the suffering the booklet told us he wasn't experiencing.

Late Tuesday night, as Geoff and I were finishing the last food I would eat before my lumpectomy the next morning, Mom called to say Dad had died. Mom had been in and out of the sunroom all day and when she came in to check on him before dinner, his breathing had stopped. She had called the coroner and my sister. Both were with her as she was speaking with me. There were no tears. Just quiet murmurs between us as I hung up and felt my grief hurtle me down the roller coaster again.

"Are you still going to have the surgery tomorrow?" Geoff asked.

"Yes."

I left Geoff to clean up the dishes and I went to bed to put an end to this very sad day.

BREAST SURGERY #1

The next morning we were up at God-knows-what-hour in order to be at Stanford by 6:00 am. This time I remembered to bring my ID with me. I was told there were a couple of "very minor procedures" they needed to do prior to the surgery to make sure they knew exactly where the tumor and the lymph nodes they wanted to remove were located.

The first procedure the doctors did was to locate the lymph nodes. They injected me with radioactive stuff that would end up in the sentinel lymph nodes (these are the first lymph nodes). It turns out that cancer flesh is the same color as healthy flesh, so doctors cannot just open you up and see what needs to be cut out (hence why the surgeon eight years prior didn't take a sample of my tumor but instead biopsied clean flesh). They need guides to help them locate the bad stuff. The radioactive stuff was injected *in my nipple*, and over the course of an hour, would make its way to my lymph nodes and stop there. The doctor would then be able to use some kind of medical version of a Geiger counter to locate the lymph nodes he should remove. I envisioned Dr. PlasticSurgeon like those guys with metal detectors looking for loose change and lost jewelry on the beach, except he was looking for radioactive lymph nodes.

And yes, you read that right. To locate the lymph nodes they needed to inject me *in my left nipple* with radioactive stuff. *Four times.* Sigh. Let me paint a crystal-clear picture for you: I was in the basement of the hospital in a room with no windows and probably a three-foot-thick door like the radiation lab because of all of the radioactive stuff they had in there – and about to inject in me. I sat on a table with both breasts just hanging there while two doctors (both male) injected me in my nipple. I think I had pants on. Who knows? I definitely had no shirt on, and like I said, I just no longer considered it weird to be naked. To be clear, getting injected in my nipple was a big freaking deal because it stung, but full-frontal nudity? No longer embarrassing.

To locate the tumor, they used a sonogram to pinpoint exactly where it was. The tumor looked like a rock cradled by fleshy waves, and the goal was to insert a wire exactly where that rock was so that Dr. PlasticSurgeon could remove the entirety of the rock and minimize the removal of the fleshy waves. Once the tumor/rock was located on the sonogram screen, they shot me with some numbing stuff and then inserted a wire into the tumor (with the other end of the wire sticking out of me). Then, to add insult to my injured breast, they then took a mammogram (yes, squished my injured breast between two cold plates and took pictures of it) so that the surgeon would have a picture of exactly where the rock and the wire were.

When I woke from the surgery, Dr. PlasticSurgeon came to see how I was feeling (great). He told me the surgery had gone well and that they had achieved "clean margins." I could go home. I was now officially cancer-free. OMFG—hurray!!! I went home to a celebratory pizza. I could see glimmers of my future from the top of this crazy roller coaster.

CHAPTER FIFTEEN

THE ROLLER COASTER THAT IS CANCER

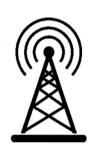

CARINGBRIDGE ENTRY: October 31, 2012

DO OVER.

So...The pathology (lab work) came back from my breast surgery and unfortunately, the surgeon didn't get "clean" margins. Eesh. So — what the hell does that mean? Well, surgeons send the tumor/flesh they have cut out to a lab and the lab looks to see if there are cancer cells near the edge of the area (the margin) the surgeon cut out. Stanford Oncology's protocol is to have a 2 cm margin that is free of cancer cells (e.g. "clean") before they declare clean margins. (My salivary gland cancer operation had "clean" margins.) What complicated things with the breast surgery is the chemotherapy I did before the surgery.

The good news is the chemotherapy worked exactly as it was supposed to – by disintegrating the tumor to a smaller size. The bad news is that as the tumor disintegrated, bits of cancer cells moved into the surrounding area and showed up in the lab work at the margins of the area cut out. So why the hell did we do the chemo before surgery (most often chemo follows surgery)? In my case, the doctors were trying to reduce the size of my tumor and get the disease out of my lymph nodes so as to simplify the surgery (and make breast conservation possible). As planned — the tumor did reduce, but the disintegration made it harder to get "clean" margins. As for the lymph nodes — the surgeon removed five lymph nodes during the initial surgery to test for disease. You may remember that the lab was going to check on them real time during the surgery – which they did – and they declared the lymph nodes free of cancer. Unfortunately, upon review of their slides, the lab determined they had been wrong and that cancer cells actually were in the first two of the five nodes. GAH! So — the first surgery was not as successful as we had initially hoped.

So what happens next? Well, I'm going in for surgery again to see if the surgeon can get more (read: all) of the cancer cells out of the tumor area. He'll do that by cutting out a larger part of the breast. He tells me that a second surgery is not all that uncommon to ensure there are clean margins – and that he has done up to four (!!) surgeries in the name of breast conservation. I told him that if we don't get it in this second surgery, I don't think we'll be discussing a third or fourth "breast conservation" surgery, but I get ahead of myself...On the lymph node front, he is considering taking out more lymph nodes – though he believes the rest of them are probably free of cancer (only the first two had disease – the other three did not). So it is a tough call. If we are conservative and remove all of the lymph nodes in the area, I will likely suffer from lymphedema (swelling of my arm due to lymphatic fluid retention) for the rest of my life; if we don't remove more lymph nodes and there is cancer *in one of them — the cancer could spread. I'm not really a fan of either scenario but am a bigger fan of my long-term HEALTH so would probably choose the lesser of the two evils — lymphedema.*

HAPPY BIRTHDAY!! *So wouldn't you know it — the next available time the surgeon has for the second surgery is MY FREAKING BIRTHDAY? Thankfully, this time instead of going in at 6:00 am for multiple tests/preparation for surgery, I get to waltz in at 1:45 pm for a 3:15 pm surgery. It is practically a spa appointment! I have been given the same instructions about food and water consumption as before — but am thrilled that I'll be able to sneak sips of water unsupervised until 1:45 pm. Whoo hoo! And you better believe I will be celebrating after surgery with unlimited birthday ice chips.*

*In other news...**I have eyebrows!!** And (some) hair! Whew. No matter how much cancer survivors who have gone through chemotherapy assure you that your hair will grow back in, there is still a nagging concern in the back of your mind that you will be THE ONE person in the history of chemotherapy whose hair doesn't grow back...So I am very happy to be on the path to hair...and so far, I think I look more Sinead O'Connor than Chia Pet, so I'm pretty happy about that.*

I'm going to take a little break from the metrics in this entry simply because I will need to adjust both the surgery metric and the overall treatment metric to reflect the additional time. Thank you for your indulgence as I shamelessly ignore these most important KPIs (key performance indicators). ☺

Thanks for all of your love and support. Xoxo Sarah & Geoff

*   *   *

CARINGBRIDGE ENTRY: November 20, 2012

ALL CLEAN.

HAPPY RE-BIRTHDAY!! *As threatened, my second breast surgery was performed on Wednesday, Nov. 7th – also known as my birthday. It all went through with much less fanfare than last surgery. I showed up at 1pm – changed into a hospital gown – waited around for the surgeon to finish his prior surgery – and then was wheeled into the operating room...No 6:00 am arrival time. No radioactive goo injected into my nipple. No wire inserted to show the doctor where he should be cutting. Nope. No one even checked to see if I had been surreptitiously drinking water...The surgeon simply used his prior incision as guide to carve a larger perimeter/ remove tissue that might still have traces of malignancy. This is a tough job for the surgeon because (as we've discussed before) cancer doesn't look any different than healthy tissue. I am told that sometimes it feels different (harder) but for the most part, he's just scooping out where the lab told him there might be additional tumor tissue – and hoping for the best. After a couple of hours I woke up — sucked on my beloved ice chips — and Geoff and I drove home to a celebratory dinner of pizza.*

Warning: I am about to talk about something gross → ***lymphatic drains.*** *Skip over this section if you get squeamish when talking about bodily functions...Okay – still with me? I wanted to share this next part with you because it's just really kind of fascinating...When I woke up after surgery #2, I discovered I had a temporary "drain" consisting of a tube coming out my side and ending in a squeezable plastic bulb where orangey-pink lymphatic fluid collects. Why a drain? Well, all told, I have had 12 lymph nodes removed.*

Lymph nodes are like bus stops along the greater lymphatic transport system. Remove lymph nodes and a big old backup of lymphatic fluid can occur – resulting in a massive traffic jam (swelling) at the place of surgery. OR the surgeon can insert a tube and fluid can be manually drained until the system figures out its new route. Or something like that. Why do I think this is so cool? Well, first I think it's super great that doctors figured out a way to allow the system to drain and not swell (much less painful and dangerous for me). And second, I think it is fascinating that the body heals itself (in general) and figures out how to redirect stuff like lymphatic fluid (in specific). So while it is a bit of a fashion bummer to have this thing poking out of me, it is helping me heal – and I am told it can be removed after Thanksgiving...So now one of the things I am thankful for this year is bulky sweaters that hide drains.

9:45 pm! The Monday night after my surgery my phone rang and caller ID told me it was Stanford. What? Who at Stanford calls at 9:45 pm? Get this: It was my surgeon calling to tell me he had just reviewed the pathology report (at 9:45 pm!?!?) and there was NO EVIDENCE OF DISEASE (NED) in any of the additional tissue or nodes he removed. Hoo-freaking-ray!!!! NOW I think I can call myself cancer-free and lucky and grateful. I can also call my hard-working surgeon a workaholic – but also a big ol' hero. Wow.

THANKSGIVING. I know I'm totally going to sound like someone with cancer here, but I feel like I have a lot to be thankful for this year. Yay. I could list a whole lot of stuff here but I think family, friends, health, and luck (oh yes – and bulky sweaters) cover most of it.

Summary metrics. They're back!

Surgery: *2 total sessions/3 completed*

150% complete! (February 7th/Oct 17th/Nov 7th). By my estimation, I have over-delivered on my surgery metric by 50%. This is bonus territory, people. If I'm in the "president's club" for cancer, I think this means I get a trip to Hawaii... Geoff, can you please confirm?

Mouth Radiation: *30 total sessions/30 completed*

100% complete! (completed May 8th)

Chemo I: *12 total sessions/12 completed*

100% complete! (completed July 23rd)

Chemo II: *4 total sessions/4 completed*

100% complete! (completed Sept 10th)

Breast Radiation: *33 total sessions/0 completed*

0% complete

Total treatment: *50 total weeks/41 completed*

82% complete (Adjusted again to reflect the new treatment timeline — estimated treatment end date of January 18th — which, ironically, is the date of my first diagnosis. Wow.)

Thanks for all of your love and support. Xoxo Sarah & Geoff

*　　*　　*

Three days after my first breast surgery (and four days after Dad's death), I was on a plane back home to help my mother make arrangements for Dad's memorial service. I felt fine—bruised, yes—but

I desperately wanted to be home. I wanted to understand how that home felt now that my Dad didn't live in it. I wanted to walk into the sunroom and feel where he had died. If my Dad's spirit was still in that space, I wanted him to know that I would cherish him and love him. And I didn't want Mom to feel alone in her house. While I don't think of her as a needy person, I also knew she had never lived alone before. She went from her parents' house to college to graduate school to living with Dad. I couldn't be with her for long, but maybe I could make the first week or two without him better.

I also wanted Death to know that I was still alive.

I did chores around the house to help her out. I cleaned out Dad's closet into helpful piles for my brother David, for Goodwill, and for trash. I smelled Dad on the clothes and wondered how long his scent would last. It's such a sappy thing in movies when characters smell the clothes of loved ones who have left and yet here I found myself smelling my Dad's much-loved Boston Red Sox sweatshirt (David pile).

At the end of that week with Mom, I stopped by the local gourmet grocery store around 8:00 pm to grab a six pack of beer. I have friends from college who moved to my hometown after graduation, and when I'm home, we gather and drink beer. Really good beer that I can only find at the gourmet grocery store in town.

So there I was in the parking lot about to head to their house when my phone rang and it said "Stanford."

"Sarah, this is Dr. PlasticSurgeon. I'm calling you because the pathology came back from your surgery last week and I'm sorry to say that we didn't achieve clean margins."

"Um. Hi, Dr. PlasticSurgeon. Um. What? Didn't pathology tell you during my surgery that everything was okay?"

"Yes. They did. But they looked again at the tissue we removed and they saw cancer cells near the edge of the tissue and in one of the lymph nodes. We're going to need to schedule you for another surgery."

No. No. NO. NO. NO! I screamed in my head. I felt myself start to go into that out-of-body experience from my first diagnosis as I processed the fact that I still had cancer in me. I just wanted this to be over. When will this be over?

As calmly as I could, I asked Dr. PlasticSurgeon when he needed me to fly back up and then set to rescheduling my flights. When I met with him two days later, he checked out my surgery site and we discussed surgery date options. His next available surgery date was November 7th. I hesitated because who wants to have surgery on your birthday? But then I thought, *Well, maybe there is something to getting your life back on your birthday?* So I took it.

I flew back down the following week for my father's memorial service. A few years earlier, at my uncle's memorial service (colon cancer), my aunt had asked my brother, sister, and me to sing an arrangement of "An Irish Blessing." As the three of us sat down after singing, my Dad leaned over to whisper to me, "I'd like you to sing that at my service some day." This was two years before his cancer had returned, but still I fiercely said to him, "I am *so* not even discussing this with you right now." When it came time to plan Dad's service with Mom, it was clear that was the song we would sing for him. So we did.

> *May the road rise up to meet you.*
> *May the wind be always at your back.*
> *May the sun shine warm upon your face;*
> *May the rains fall soft upon your fields and until we meet again,*
> *May God hold you in the palm of His hand.*

Dad didn't believe in God, so much of the ceremony of his service was for those in the audience who did. But he would have loved that song.

BREAST SURGERY #2 (or three if you count the first 2004 biopsy)

There was a lot less fanfare with the second breast surgery – thank God! Geoff and I again trekked down to Stanford though this time for a leisurely 1:00 pm date with the knife. I was told there was no need to do all of the tests/scans/fanfare to identify where my tumor was. The surgeon would carve out a larger perimeter around where my tumor had been by simply using his prior incisions as guides.

When I awoke from that surgery, I was surprised to discover a tube sticking out of my side called a "lymphatic drain."

I was not prepared for a lymphatic drain. I had not read about lymphatic drains, nor had anyone spoken to me about this being a possible outcome of this surgery. It was just *there* when I woke up.

I was told the drain would be in place for a week or two while my body re-routed its lymphatic system (*What*!? The body just *does* that!?) and then the medical staff could pull it out of me. I was given a piece of paper with columns and dates where I was meant to record the amount of fluid I found (and expunged) from my drain every day. Very helpfully, the piece of paper had room for three weeks' worth of data collection, which I knew I wouldn't need because I would only have this drain in me for a week or two. A week or two which ended up being six. Long. Weeks. Of. Drain.

How is it to have six weeks of a plastic tube sticking out of you, you ask?

Well, first of all, there is an "ick" factor. There is sticky, pinkish fluid that is dripping out of you all day long. How do I know it is sticky? Because on more than one occasion I managed to spill it while trying to expunge and measure it, which *totally* messed up the data I was asked to track by my doctor. Multiple times a day, I measured the amount of lymphatic fluid I was generating—physical proof as the liquid lessened that my system was rerouting itself—so the doctor could okay the ripping of the drain out of me.

Second, the tube and drain hang down the side of your body like a big, lumpy bungee cord that would just go on swinging unchecked if you didn't safety-pin it to your bra or t-shirt. The bummer about the safety-pinning of the drain is that the big, swinging bungee cord running down the side of your body becomes a bigger lumpy-lump on the side of you that is tricky to hide. Thankfully for me, it was November when I had the drain and bulky sweaters didn't look out of place.

Beyond the unsightliness of a bungee cord attached to you, why would you bother to safety-pin it up? Because if you don't, that damned tube is going to get caught on the most unlikely things—like the handle on your gadget drawer in your kitchen. A small tug on the drain isn't a big deal at all, but when you are making a quick move in the kitchen (to remove a boiling pot of pasta from the stove or grab a towel to take a cookie sheet from the oven, for example), that is when the drain will catch on the drawer pull. That quick yank on the drain will cause a primordial jabbing pain originating somewhere in the internal lady parts—thus well worth avoiding. So safety-pin it to my bra I did.

I was patient for the first couple of weeks with the drain. It was kind of a novelty and as I said, it was November and the sweaters I wore helped to hide the awkward bulkiness of the drain under my armpit. But then November turned into December and even though I was still only sporting peach fuzz on my head, I wanted desperately to go to holiday parties wearing little black dresses or sparkly tops with short skirts—neither of which looked especially good with medical plastic awkwardly swinging next to me.

When I finally was allowed to have the drain removed, it was five days before Geoff and I were leaving for Punta Mita, Mexico for a last tropical getaway before I would return to work in January. The nurse took hold of the tube and asked "Are you ready?" I nodded yes and braced myself for the primordial jabbing pain...It hurt, yes—but not nearly as much as I had feared. In fact, my fear was that the skin surrounding the tube had actually started to grow into the tube somehow and we wouldn't be able to remove it. Once the tube was out, I shared that fear with the nurse now holding my disembodied lymphatic drain. She started laughing and said "Oh my God—when you took your shirt off and I saw your drain and learned how long it had been in you, I had the same fear!" *Thank God* my skin decided to let go of that drain.

I'VE GOT A CRUSH ON YOU

Living in Northern California it seems cliché to say you have a friend who is a winemaker. However, one of the most wonderful friendships Geoff brought to our relationship is the one he has with James, an *amazing* winemaker in Healdsburg, located in Sonoma County. I have often said to Geoff that being friends with a winemaker must be a little like developing a friendship with a drug dealer. And while it has been challenging for our wallets and our waistlines, the depth of the friendship has more than made up for it in the nourishment of our souls. We love James and his wife, Kerry.

One of the reasons it is so easy to love James and Kerry is that they are so humble about their craft and so open to sharing it with the people in their lives. James patiently explains how he makes his wine while Kerry generously pours wine into my glass. They invite us to parties with their winemaker friends, and Geoff and I do our best to attend every time.

Beyond parties, we are invited most years to participate in Crush as members of the MOG squad. MOG stands for "materials other than grapes," and it refers to the work harvesters and winemakers do to remove materials other than grapes from the bins of grapes that will go into the presser to make the wine. "Crush," also known as Harvest, is the time in winemaking when the grapes are picked and the winemaking process begins. It generally starts in late August and can go on through November, depending on the weather and the type of grapes you are harvesting.

The MOG process consists of someone (often James or Thomas, another amazing winemaker who often helps James) driving a forklift with a bin of grapes up to a machine that looks like a big funnel. The bin of grapes is then dumped into the funnel and onto a conveyor belt where MOGers like me stand in rain boots (it is a wet, sticky business) and a red t-shirt (or something you don't mind staining) with a hat and lots of sunscreen to protect you from the punishing sun. For ten years plus, I have picked out leaves, mildewed grapes, unripe grapes, pincher bugs, a praying mantis, water bottles, and batteries—all from the conveyor belt of grapes, and all in service of purifying the substance that will make the glorious elixir called wine.

You can't predict when the grapes will be ready. It is the decision of the winemaker when to pick, but once picked, those grapes need to be processed to start the winemaking. My contribution to the process ends once I step away from the conveyor belt, but it is really fun to think that you're helping in some small way to create this beautiful product. Most years I have only been able to participate in 1 or 2 days (mostly weekends) of MOGing, but in 2012, I was able to join every day of Harvest because my chemo treatments just kinda lined up to allow me to do so. Yay.

Day one started at 8:00 am with shots of tequila for everyone there to help. I stepped right up and grabbed my shot glass, confident that my blood labs would indicate to the doctor if my liver couldn't handle it. I put on extra sunscreen and stood under an umbrella that Kerry had placed over us, as I knew I would be especially sensitive to the sun given my chemo. We probably processed six tons of grapes that day and earned the lunch of pizza and ice cream Kerry gave us.

Thomas, who had been working the forklift that day, pulled me to the side to tell me, "Sarah, I had cancer too. In my leg. I just wanted you to know. I survived." I was stunned by his news and so grateful that he shared it with me. And while he couldn't promise me that I would survive, his eyes told me I would.

The next day more than enough MOGers showed up to help, and James and Kerry pulled me to the side to ask if I could help them with another project. Kerry walked me into their wine cellar—which was roughly the size of a small bedroom—and asked if I could organize it for them. As someone who loves to bring order to chaos, this was a dream. I organized by winery, by wine type, by vintage...and entered all of it into a spreadsheet so that James and Kerry could keep track of it. They even had me create a wall called the "grab wall" of wines that needed to be drunk soon so they knew what to "grab next."

I had always loved James and Kerry and the people they surround themselves with, but this Harvest was especially meaningful to me. After a day or two of answering questions about my cancer, we just fell in to talking about the things we would normally talk about, like politics or the music we were listening to or the newest restaurant we had been to. I felt normal. I felt needed. I felt I had a purpose.

I felt ready to re-enter my wonderful life.

CHAPTER SIXTEEN

SPEAKING OF CANCER...

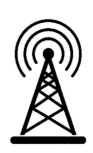

CARINGBRIDGE ENTRY: Jan 11, 2013

HI HO! HI HO!

It's back to work I go! *I really **could not** be happier to be returning to work and getting my life back to some kind of normal. **This Monday**, January 14th, I will return to work at eBay – 52 weeks after I left. Yup – 52 weeks! A full year. Who knew that cancer fighting could take a full year? Certainly not me. When (in June) the insurance company asked me to ask the oncologist to project how long I would be out on disability, the doctor said I should be excused from work until March 2013. I looked at the doctor and sputtered incredulously "MARCH? No, no, no – you must have that wrong. I've mapped out my treatment plan and if everything goes as scheduled, I should be back at work by the end of November...just after Thanksgiving..."*

*Are you one of those people who (like me) is just SO AMAZED when you get something just **totally** wrong? I mean – like MONTHS wrong?*

To review: *October/November was the whole three MRI fiasco/"Lite-Brite" potential-new-chemo-resistant-lump-scare/core biopsy showing new lump was benign/ breast surgery #1/not clean margins/breast surgery #2/introduction of lymphatic drain/and (finally!) clean margins. Remember all of that? Well, the important part to remember is the CLEAN MARGINS thing. After three surgeries (one mouth, two breast), we believe the cancer is out of me. Whew!*

But you know what wasn't out of me? *That fascinating (some might say f***ing) lymphatic drain. You might remember me describing the drain as a way to relieve fluid and pressure while my body figured out how to remap my lymphatic transportation system. Well, my body took its freaking time to do so. The doctors (and nurses, and physicians' assistants, and even one woman at a holiday party who confided in me that she had had a boob job ten years ago) assured me that drains generally stay in for a week. One week.* ***Maybe*** *two. How long did my lymphatic team take to figure it out?* ***Six*** *weeks.* ***During the holidays —*** *when a big bulb doesn't exactly accessorize with a little black dress. Honestly, it got to the point where my body was healing so well around the tube (good job, skin!) that I thought the drain was going to be a permanent part of me. When it actually came time to remove the tube, the nurse admitted to me afterward that she was more than a little nervous to tug it out...but thankfully, out it came on December 14th. Just in time for....*

The Presidents' Club trip to Puerto Vallarta, Mexico!! *Whoo hoo! Post-drain removal, we were told it would be 2-3 weeks before I could begin radiation in order for my body*

to heal. Geoff (realizing I had qualified for a trip due
to my "exceeds most" rating on my metrics) started
scouting out flights **anywhere warm** for the week before
Christmas. Puerto Vallarta (PV) is a 3.5-hour (relatively
cheap) flight from SF and off we went!! And I was a good
kid and sat under the umbrella with sunblock 50 slathered
all over me. I mean – what do I want with a third cancer
(trifecta, anyone)? It would be downright greedy...And I am
happy to report it was a delightful five days away that felt
much longer.

Speaking of longer...My hair is longer. Yes, besides eyebrows
and eyelashes – I now have (gray) hair!! Did I know it would
grow back in gray? (Most common question) to which I
answer "UM. OF COURSE! I have been dyeing it for ten
years!" Is it curlier than it was? Well, it is most certainly
curly – in fact, my dear brother's reaction was "You kind of
look like a labradoodle," which is actually a better description
than my own, as I was describing it as "the Brillo pad on my
head." So I think "labradoodle" is a step up, actually. I would
tell you that – living in San Francisco – I do look like I'm about
to go protest something at any moment.

So where do we go from here? The next step is 30 rounds
of radiation to my left breast – followed by five years of a
hormone therapy drug called tamoxifen that will block the
estrogen and progesterone my breast cancer apparently liked
to feast on. And – for the foreseeable future — I will do scans
(MRI, CT or PET) every six months to both the head/neck and
the breasts to ensure nothing is going on. But mostly, from
here I am hoping to get back to living my life as normally as
possible. Wanna help me with that? ☺ Good – because I
count on each of you. xoxo

Summary metrics. Ooooh! I am SO CLOSE to finished!!!

Surgery: 2 total sessions/3 completed — *150% complete! (February 7th/Oct 17th/Nov 7th).*

Mouth Radiation: 30 total sessions/30 completed — *100% complete! (completed May 8th)*

Chemo I: 12 total sessions/12 completed — *100% complete! (completed July 23rd)*

Chemo II: 4 total sessions/4 completed — *100% complete! (completed Sept 10th)*

Breast Radiation: 30 total sessions/3 completed — *10% complete*

Total treatment: 55 total weeks/48 completed — *87% complete (Adjusted again to reflect the new treatment timeline with revised end date of February 26th, 2013.)*

Thanks for all of your love and support. Xoxo Sarah & Geoff

*   *   *

CARINGBRIDGE ENTRY: March 20, 2013

ALL METRICS NOW AT 100%!

*Hi! I can tell when it's time for me to post again because I have all you metrics junkies following up with me via phone and email. Thank you. And — of course — I have some pretty BIG news. Tuesday February 26th was my last day of radiation as well as my last day of **active** cancer treatment. The tech team at Stanford celebrated by giving me a certificate indicating I had completed the full course* *of radiation required. I celebrated by baking chocolate chip cookies for the technicians, the valet parking guys, and the administrative team in the oncology department — all of whom were rooting for me — just like you. Yay! Then Geoff and I went out to breakfast and other than that, it was a pretty low-key day. I went into work, went to some meetings, talked with colleagues about work-related topics, and went home in a totally-normal-workday kind of way. And you know what? It was* **perfect**. *I have returned to my normal life and I could not be happier about that.*

So — what is it like being back to work?

Well, it is an adjustment — but in a good way. It took me such a very long time to unplug from work initially after my diagnosis. In fact, at one point my HR colleague turned off my access to email so that I would stop checking it. Wow! The truth is that in the early days of cancer diagnosis, email was a welcome reprieve from thinking about the bigger issues going on in my life. Now that I am back at work, I have been surprised how quickly I have plugged right back in...And I like to think that while I'm still very much the same person — maybe I've slowed down a little and have more perspective.

Like coffee. I've been back to work six weeks now — and I've arranged to "grab coffee" with multiple people to re-establish our connections and come up to speed on just what the hell has been going on over the past year. For the first three days of my return to work, I was averaging five coffees a day before I realized that this just wasn't sustainable. I was positively vibrating from all of the caffeine in me. I am out of practice — and had forgotten that "coffee" is more of an excuse to get up from your desk — as certainly no one is expected to consume five cups of coffee a day even in the name of keeping appearances.

What does the future (treatment) look like?

*Well, as I said above, the "active" treatment part is over except for some hormone therapy I'll be taking for the next five years. I'll be taking a drug called tamoxifen which is meant to block the estrogen and progesterone hormones. Other than that — we wait and we monitor — with the hope that neither of these buggers returns. Both the head and neck team and the breast team want to do scans/tests every 3-6 months for the next five years. After that, we'll likely go once a year. The **good** news is that both cancers were slow growing/non-aggressive — so if there is a recurrence — we should hopefully have time on our side. And for that (and for so many other reasons), I feel very lucky.*

Summary metrics. *I am happy to report that ALL metrics now stand at 100% (or better).*

Surgery: *2 (planned) sessions/3 completed* *150% complete! (February 7th/ Oct 17th/Nov 7th).*

Mouth Radiation: *30 total sessions/30 completed* *100% complete! (completed May 8th)*

Chemo I: *12 total sessions/12 completed* *100% complete! (completed July 23rd)*

Chemo II: *4 total sessions/4 completed* *100% complete! (completed Sept 10th)*

Breast Radiation: *33 total sessions/33 completed* *100% complete (completed Feb 26th)*

Total treatment: *55 total weeks/55 completed* 100% complete

End of treatment = end of blog.

I think/hope/believe this will be my last blog post given that active cancer treatment is over. I am celebratory and joyous and thankful that I am on the other side of the mountain — yet it's kind of weird after so much blogging to just stop it. While the subject was sometimes challenging for me — it was a chance to share broadly what was going on with me physically and emotionally — and to get an almost immediate "atta girl!" from many of you. That "atta girl" was more helpful than my pride would like to admit — and went a long way toward making this journey easier. **Thank you.**

A dear friend I made over the past year was diagnosed with breast cancer last week. She sent out an email to her support network detailing the weeks and myriad of tests she had been undergoing while her doctors came to her diagnosis. I cried with the memory of my own first few weeks of living with the knowledge I had cancer — not knowing what the outcome would be. My friend was diagnosed early — and she and her doctors are treating it aggressively — but it is an uncertain time. I am hopeful to be helpful to her on her journey — as she has been on mine — if only just to hold her hand and say "I know..." And isn't that what our lives are all about? Holding one another's hand as we each make our own journey. Whew! Heavy way to end this whole blog business...but true to how I'm feeling.

Thank you so much to all of you for your love and support over the past year. *Did I mention that I feel lucky? Well, I do. I am rich beyond what I can comprehend in love from friends and family. Thank you. Xoxo Sarah & Geoff*

*   *   *

SPEAKING ABOUT CANCER

Once the most physically obvious parts of my treatment were complete (the radiation that created the mouth sores, the chemo-induced hair loss, the mofo lymphatic drain from the surgeries), I wanted to get back to work. I think, similar to when I was initially diagnosed, I wanted to get back to my normal life as quickly as I could. I wanted to get into the familiar rhythm of working—to have a schedule and a place I needed to be every day. I wanted to feel like I was still contributing, like I was needed.

To his ongoing credit, Devin told me there was no rush for me to come back. "Come back when you're ready," he told me. "But I *am* ready," I insisted. So I pushed Devin and Kristin on my return date and they agreed I could come back in January into my old role as chief of staff. So on a Monday in mid-January, I returned to work almost a year to the day after I had left.

I was so eager to get back to normal life that I didn't spend a lot of time thinking about what re-entry would look like. I wanted to slip back into my working life without acknowledging I had been gone for the past year. Like maybe the fact that I was 35 pounds lighter and had short curly gray hair growing slowly out of my head wasn't obvious and we could all just pretend like it hadn't happened? As a result, I didn't think through how I would field questions like, "Where have you been?" or "Wow! Bold new haircut?" or, if they knew what had been going on, "How are you *doing*?"

After a year of blogging and speaking regularly and openly with family, friends, and any medical professional who would listen about cancer, I was surprised to find myself getting choked up when a colleague would ask. It was as if there was this raw nerve just at the surface of my unconscious that I kept touching. I thought I had fully processed my cancer diagnosis and had healed both physically and emotionally.

But there it was—this raw nerve that stung my eyes and gave me mini panic attacks as I struggled to find the right words to describe what had happened and how I was doing.

Just as I had done with my initial message to friends, I developed a set of talking points I could fall back on that addressed my year of cancer at a high level. At a ten-thousand-foot level, I could impartially hit the highlights and avoid diving into the more dangerous subjects like how I really was doing. Because I wasn't doing well. Physically, I had come out the other side of my year of cancer treatments—but emotionally, I was still battling. I wasn't "over" cancer like I thought I was. I could say cancer out loud but I was still (still!?) processing what had just happened. I was shell-shocked. And if I am honest, I was still scared.

GOING REALLY PUBLIC ABOUT CANCER

After I returned to work, two work friends of mine, Anne and Kate, asked me if I would be willing to talk about my cancer diagnosis at a management training day they were hosting for the leaders of StubHub. They wanted to challenge the leaders to think about the level of intimacy and empathy they were showing with their teammates and those who reported to them. They hoped that by my speaking publicly about what could be an awkward work situation – they could challenge these people managers to think deeply about how to lead with empathy and human-ness.

At the time, eBay owned StubHub but they operated separately. Occasionally talent (people) would be traded between companies – but it didn't happen often, so I probably only knew about five of the 150 people there that day. For most in the room, I was a stranger. Anne and Kate asked that I share at a high level my eBay work history leading up to my appointment as chief of staff, and then give detail about the day of my diagnosis and how I shared that diagnosis with my manager (Devin) and with the wider executive team. Then they would open up the room for folks to ask me questions if I was open to that. I agreed to do the talk but warned them both there was a good chance talking about it so publicly might trigger tears – though I would do my best to keep it together.

Turns out, I didn't cry. (Go me!) But a number of folks in the room did. As I told my story, I told them what it felt like to tell my manager (Devin) and my HR business partner (Kristin) I had cancer. I told them of Devin telling me to go home and not come back until I was better. I told them about Cancer Island and how cut off from other living humans I felt after my diagnosis, but that Kristin (and Dr. Fertility) had texted me all weekend, giving me a lifeline from Cancer Island.

As I answered questions I scanned the room and noticed a number of people (4? 5?) bending over their laps or shielding their eyes. Then I watched two different people leave the room. I was curious as I watched them leave, as I hadn't shared any particularly gut-wrenching details of my diagnosis or my treatment. In fact, I had tried to keep my stories funny and light—much as I had done in my blog. And, I reasoned, these people didn't *know me*. There was no reason for my story to bring tears to them.

Then it dawned on me...it wasn't me. These folks weren't reacting to *my* story. Rather, each of these people had been touched by cancer (whether it was their own, a friend's or a family member's) currently or in the past, and talking so openly about it was bringing those other experiences into the room for them. It was not something I had anticipated in talking so publicly about my diagnosis. My primary concern was whether *I* would be able to keep it together; I hadn't thought about how my story might touch the raw nerves of others in the room.

I was mobbed by people after the talk. The comments fell into roughly four categories. Many people wanted to tell me how brave they thought I was to speak so publicly about cancer – that it felt like a private topic for people – not one covered in a corporate training program. They wondered aloud what other topics I could speak with them about! I appreciated their enthusiasm and told them so. Several people wanted to tell me how I helped them laugh about a topic they had previously been afraid to broach with others – which was also great to hear. I, of course, love being told I'm funny. A number of people managers thanked me for sharing what it was like to be an employee going through a crisis as they felt I had helped them think differently about how they might be a more empathetic manager. (YAY! That is what Anne and Kate hoped they would accomplish with this talk!) The last group of people were where I spent the most time. These were the audience members who actually had an employee or family member or friend who was going through cancer treatments. With these people, I spoke about how hard it must be for them – and how cancer (or other life-threatening diseases) impacts everyone around it. I promised to be a resource to them if they needed to talk more.

I was unbelievably energized by the experience. When Anne and Kate asked if I would repeat the talk for the StubHub people managers in Connecticut – I could not say YES! fast enough. Anne and Kate expanded the next training into a full day session and I had the opportunity to facilitate a couple of breakout sessions. It. Was. Awesome. I was so excited that my story was so *useful* to the managers I spoke with during those two training sessions. Kate and I brainstormed other future topics beyond Empathy I might be able to speak to like *How to show up as a manager* or *How to talk about tough topics* or *How to build Resiliency*, etc. On my own I started to think about topics I could speak with groups of doctors and/or patients about like *Self-Advocacy: How to project manage your doctors / your care* or *How to talk with friends and family about your cancer.*

This experience helped me realize the profound impact I could have on others by speaking openly and honestly about my cancer experience.

I vowed to not shy away from any other public speaking opportunity presented to me. I thought again about the book I had started writing about my cancer experience – could that have a positive impact on people too?

MY TO-DO LIST

I have a personal to-do list that I keep on my computer but also print out so I can keep track of all of the things I want to do. This is a tactical list—not a bucket list—so I have items like the gathering of our tax documents and the need to send thank yous listed on the to-do list. I also have started to keep track of when I need to schedule my doctor's appointments so I don't forget to schedule them. (Next head & neck MRI: next January.) I've broken the to-do list into two sections: Shorter-term to-dos are on the front side of the page. Longer-term to-dos occupy the back side. Longer-term to-dos include the need to make an earthquake/fire plan or the list of photo albums I want to create.

Also on the longer-term to-do list is a catalog of friends who have or had cancer who I want to check in with regularly. I also have a list of friends whose partners died from cancer. If the person currently has cancer, I try to text them every week to check in on the progress of treatments. It is my way of providing that lifeline to Cancer Island that I received the first weekend of my diagnosis from Dr. Fertility and from Kristin. I want them to know that someone is actively thinking of them. I want to proactively be within text-reach to answer any questions they have. I want to assure them any feelings or fears they're having are valid. I want them to know they're not alone.

If the person is no longer being treated, I try to text or call or email every other month or so. I don't want to overwhelm or become their little cancer reminder. ("Hi! It's February—how's your cancer?") I just want to check in. I send a quick note to let them know I am thinking of them. Most times these dear friends just send a heart emoji back acknowledging

I have texted and sending love back my way. I want them to know that I understand cancer doesn't end when treatments end. After treatments end, there are follow-up scans and tests and check-ins you have to keep track of. After treatments end, there are little aches and pains that are probably associated with growing older (lucky us) but which the cancer survivor can invest quality time imagining are a recurrence. I want them to know I haven't left their side. I am still walking this cancer journey with them, wherever it takes us.

CHAPTER SEVENTEEN

LIVING WITH CANCER

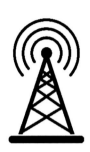

WHY AM I STILL ALIVE?

When I started writing this chapter, I removed a name from my to-do list. Her name was Sarvenaz. I met her at work in probably 2010? She would have been about 30 then. In the highly collaborative culture of eBay, Sarvenaz was an outlier. It wasn't that she was actively confrontational but she wasn't afraid to ask very direct questions—even if it made things uncomfortable in the room. I remember gaping at a bold question she once put to an executive, flinching at her directness while also impressed by her daring. She had questions and she asked them. Sarvenaz died at age 39 from metastatic breast cancer.

Sarvenaz was diagnosed in 2016, four years after me. Like me, she took a leave of absence from eBay to do her treatments and returned to work with a very short pixie cut. Unlike me, she went out on leave a year later when her cancer returned.

When the corporate grapevine reached me that Sarvenaz was on leave again, I sent her an email to offer myself as a resource. We met for lunch.

I told Sarvenaz my cancer story and shyly admitted that I had started writing a book about it. I told her I wanted the book to be poignant and true but also funny where I could be funny. She told me she felt it was important to tell *all* of the stories about cancer, to touch on the pain and terror of it, in addition to the sometimes ridiculous indignities of the disease. She asked to read it and promised to be honest in her feedback.

She shared her diagnosis story. She shared her frustration when she suspected her cancer had returned, but she couldn't seem to convince her doctors to run the scans. I listened to her brave acceptance that by the time they did the scans the cancer had spread to her brain. I was apoplectic when she told me this. She now had a stage four breast cancer diagnosis, which has a 25% survival rate five years from diagnosis. I raged. I cursed. How had the doctors not listened to her!? Why didn't they run the tests and catch the cancer before it could reach her brain!? Knowing these reactions didn't change anything, I simply started crying helplessly at the table as she calmly nodded at me and said, "I know."

When I read the message that Sarvenaz had died, I immediately wanted to find our last email, our last text exchange to find evidence of our connection—to touch the time when she was alive. I remembered our last lunch in San Francisco, when we had gone to a makeup boutique in the Fillmore District shopping for fake eyelashes because hers were now gone. Our last lunch was in June. Our last email exchange, in September. My unanswered texts in November, December, last Wednesday.

I stood at my computer scrolling through pictures of Sarvenaz on Facebook. Childhood pictures. Pictures holding her daughter, looking up at her husband, laughing. I swatted at the tears flowing down my face as I cried. I looked up toward the ceiling to stop them from running down my nose. I pressed my hands against my eyes to push the tears back and cool my eyelids. I tried to slow my breathing and stifle the sobs that were bubbling out of me. Geoff walked up behind me and hugged me around my waist, rocking with me as the tears came. I wasn't a close friend of Sarvenaz's. I was a colleague with whom she happened to share this awful common bond of breast cancer. But I mourned her loss. She was smart and funny and was in love with her husband and little girl. It was just so unfair.

Why did I live and Sarvenaz did not? Michelle (melanoma). Tim (brain). Simon (bowel). Peter (lung). Trista (melanoma). Sarvenaz (breast). These are the names of friends who have had cancer and died within the last ten years of my life, two of whom were diagnosed and died since I was diagnosed. Really good people, all of them. Why did I live when these other friends did not? Why? I am no better or deserving than any of them were. Cancer is so random and so unrelenting and so unfair.

When I was first diagnosed I remember thinking how I had just married my love. A year and a half later I couldn't die from cancer, could I? But Michelle and Tim both died within a year of marrying the loves of their too-short lives. Peter had a three-year-old daughter. Sarvenaz's daughter was six.

What I feel isn't survivor's guilt. I don't feel unworthy of surviving cancer. I am grateful I survived cancer. I am grateful I get more time in this world with the people I love. What I feel is grief/sadness/loss for these friends who didn't get more time. I mourn how very unfair it is for their loves.

Why? Why? Why?

SURROGACY

After two years of good news checkups, I began to believe that I might live and Geoff and I revisited the idea of having a child. As a child of the seventies, I grew up on Schoolhouse Rock and without question, the song written for the number three is my standout favorite:

"A man and a woman had a little baby—yes, they did! Yes, they did! There were three in the family...it's a magic number."

While I was so grateful for this wonderful life I was still living with Geoff, I couldn't help wondering if it would be made more magical if there was a baby in it. I felt greedy and slightly ashamed that I was demanding this in my life. Shouldn't I just be happy and grateful that I had survived cancer (for now) and be satisfied?

We had those 16 embryos just sitting on ice at the Stanford Fertility Center and they began to burn a hole in my uterus. Why pay the storage fees, why not donate them to research, if we weren't going to use them?

In 2015, two years after my cancer treatments ended, we returned to the office we had frequented in 2010 and 2011 for fertility treatments, but this time we met with the nurses to discuss surrogates and how we might go about identifying one. We discussed fees and legal issues—and we started girding ourselves emotionally for what might lie ahead.

About this same time, I had my two-years-since-treatment checkup with my breast oncologist, Dr. BreastOnc. The two-year checkup is a big deal/milestone with breast cancer. Getting to your two-, five-, and ten-year anniversaries post-breast cancer are big reasons to celebrate. At the end of this appointment, as we were all smiling and celebrating this first milestone, it occurred to me to tell Dr. BreastOnc that Geoff and I were contemplating a baby.

"You know, two years out I'm starting to believe that I might live. And with that confidence, Geoff and I are talking with Dr. Fertility about finding a surrogate for our embryos."

Dr. BreastOnc looked surprised but then quickly added, "That is terrific news and I'm so glad you brought this up...because I was just reading a study from Europe, where they have socialized medicine and can therefore follow the medical records of patients pretty easily. In Belgium and Germany, the researchers found that there were a number of women who had had breast cancer—and were on tamoxifen—but who willfully stopped taking tamoxifen (against their doctor's advice) in order to become pregnant. They had babies and went back on the tamoxifen after they finished breastfeeding. What the research tracked and concluded was that these women did *not* have higher incidences of recurrence of breast cancer."

I held my breath and waited for Dr. BreastOnc to tell me that this couldn't work for me. But she just stood there smiling at me so I asked, "Wait. What are you saying? Are you saying I could go off tamoxifen, have a baby, and go back on after—and not have a higher chance of recurrence?"

"That is what the research would seem to indicate. We would obviously follow you very closely during your pregnancy, but I would be supportive of you trying to get pregnant if you'd like to try it."

I waited to speak with Geoff about this until we both got home that night.

His first response was, "I want a guarantee that the cancer won't come back. I don't want anything that we do to encourage or cause the cancer to come back. I want guarantees. If we can't get guarantees, I don't want to do it. I don't want to endanger your life. We can use a surrogate or we can *not* have a child at all. Your life is more important than this."

Wow—such a fiercely loyal and loving husband have I. But guarantees were not something we would ever have with either of these cancers.

"Sweetheart. Unfortunately, we will never have a guarantee that these cancers won't recur regardless of whether I pursue a pregnancy. These cancers are motherf***ers. They could come back at any time, especially the salivary gland cancer, which we know is incurable. Yes, absolutely the challenge with pregnancy is all of the hormones, as my breast cancer was fueled by estrogen and progesterone...but Dr. BreastOnc will follow my pregnancy and check in on me regularly. If we find something, we will get after it immediately."

We spent the next three months discussing whether I should pursue a pregnancy. Yup. Three months. Now when I say "three months discussing," this doesn't mean that we discussed this all the time or even every day. Our marital style of discussing topics is to lob a few comments at one another during a drive somewhere or a hike, and then we go off and think about it individually until the next drive or hike. So it was kind of like an ongoing discussion for three months with no real definitive end.

Beyond Geoff's "I want a guarantee that you won't get cancer again," neither of us could think of a reason we didn't want to pursue a pregnancy. Yes, I recognized that either cancer could come back, but it also might not. And given I had survived the treatments from the first two cancers, I became very optimistic that should either recur, we could cut it out with surgery, burn it up with radiation, and/or flush it out with chemotherapy. In many ways, I think deciding to have a child is one of the most optimistic decisions we make as human beings and I was feeling pretty optimistic.

And what I kept coming back to is how much I had always wanted to be pregnant. I wanted to watch *my body* change as the pregnancy progressed and took over *my body*. I wanted to know what it felt like to have a baby kick inside me. I wanted to give birth. I wanted to experience all of that and if I was being told by my oncologist that we could try...I wanted to try.

But to do so, I was going to have to go off tamoxifen, which was my only current defense against breast cancer. I had heard girlfriends who were on tamoxifen like me talk about how sometimes they would forget to take their daily pill. "I just take it when I remember." Wow. That was not me *at all*. I was diligent about taking my tamoxifen each and every day, and the idea that I would stop was a little chilling to me. But if I wanted to get pregnant, I needed to trust that I would be okay without it and, like the brave Belgian and German women before me, I would start it up again post-pregnancy and have no recurrence. I had to believe this was possible.

So I did. I stopped taking tamoxifen in May, and by early August I was taking all of the estrogen and progesterone patches, supplements, and shots needed to prepare my body for an embryo transfer. We hadn't had a chance to do an actual embryo transfer when we had gone through fertility treatments in 2010-2011, so this was a new process for us. And it was quick —like 20 minutes tops!

The funniest part of the transfer day was that I undressed, got on the table, and as we waited for Dr. Fertility to come to the room to do the transfer, another doctor (geneticist? embryologist?) came into the room and asked "So...how many embryos are we transferring today?"

What!?

"Um, one! Only one! Please only do one!"

That threw us for a moment. Apparently the fertility center had unfrozen a number of our embryos to see which one was of the highest quality, and many couples will choose to transfer a couple of embryos with the hope that one will take. But we hoped this first transfer would work—and if it didn't, we would consider multiple embryos at the next transfer.

I wasn't very optimistic about this first transfer. I knew I was infertile from our two years of fertility treatments. Granted, we had an egg donor, but I was 47 at this point, well past the age many consider to be too old for a pregnancy. And I wasn't sure if a body that had fought so hard to not die could transfer those skills to create life. But Geoff had agreed I could have this one try at pregnancy. If it didn't work, then perhaps that was The Universe telling us I wasn't meant to carry a child. If it didn't work, I would go back on tamoxifen and resume my fabulous life and we would go back to discussing whether a surrogate was the next logical step.

But...I got pregnant!

I had three months of nausea. I don't know what they're talking about when they say "*morning* sickness," as it was really "*all-day* sickness" that I experienced. I sucked ginger lozenges and ate freeze-dried green beans— the only thing that could hold off the nausea but not fill me up, which caused greater nausea—like it was my job. I actually lost weight in the first trimester.

Based upon Dr. Fertility's recommendation, I sought pregnancy care at the medical center that had originally misdiagnosed my breast cancer and had diagnosed my salivary gland cancer with Dr. Maxillofacial's jarring phone call. This was a true leap of faith and one of intentional forgiveness. I know that sounds kind of dramatic, but even though I knew no doctor had intentionally misdiagnosed me and that it wasn't Dr. Maxillofacial's fault I had adenoid cystic carcinoma, I was still kind of mad about those two experiences. But I told myself that gynecology is separate from obstetrics, and that the obstetrics team probably didn't even know the people in the head and neck department. (And if they *did* know them, they wouldn't like them either.) This would be a different experience and it would be fine.

And it was.

My body loved being pregnant. I didn't love the whole not-drinking-alcohol thing, but once I was nauseated, I didn't want to drink anything anyway, and then I just kind of got out of the habit. I encouraged Geoff to keep drinking but even his drinking dropped off when he didn't have a partner in crime.

I visited the hospital weekly so the doctors could track the progress of my pregnancy. Given it was a teaching hospital, I met with many doctors – all of whom were fascinated by my unusual? obscure? medical history. I was asked detailed questions each visit – my answers eliciting responses like "Oh wow" and "You're kidding me" and "wow, that is a lot."

- Petit Mal epilepsy from age 2-14.
- Patella-ectomy at 12.
- Deep vein thrombosis at 36.
- Adenoid Cystic Carcinoma diagnoses at 44.
- Invasive Ductal Carcinoma diagnosis at 44.
- Pregnant at 47.

These visits were paired with chidings by the nurses to gain more weight. I argued I was eating healthfully and wasn't holding back. My body just didn't seem to want or need to gain a lot of weight. The baby was definitely on the low end of the weight scale, but the doctor wasn't concerned.

In my 37th week, the nurses started telling me the baby should start turning down—heading toward the birth canal. But this baby...well, it loved lodging its head just under my ribcage on the right. The doctor told me if it didn't move, they were going to have to do an "external cephalic version."

What the *hell* is that?

Apparently, an external cephalic version is when doctors manually (externally) manipulate the baby by pushing its feet or buttocks in order to turn the baby down into the birth canal. But seriously, in thousands of years of child birthing has no doctor come up with a different way of turning the baby outside of brute force? I did read some website that gave me yoga poses to do that would encourage the baby to flip, but that didn't work either. So "version" it was...

It was totally, completely medieval. Two doctors got on either side of me and pushed opposite ways to try to reorient the baby. The first time they did it (week 38), the baby was still relatively small (5-ish pounds), and while it was uncomfortable, it was okay.

In week 39, I had two sonogram appointments. On Tuesday of that week, the baby was head down, ready for birth. On Thursday, it had flipped again and was in its favorite position just under my rib cage. *Gah.* The nurses started talking about admitting me early to the hospital (that day!) to have another "version." I promised them that I was scheduled to check in to the hospital in order to be induced on the following Monday. Couldn't I go home for the weekend and just check in on Monday? After some back and forth and my best Jedi mind tricks ("We've already done one version and the baby flipped. Who knows if the baby will flip again? If it does, couldn't we do a version on Monday?"), the nurses let me go home.

Because...OMFG, I wasn't ready to go to the hospital. I hadn't filled out my birth plan. I didn't have my hospital bag. I didn't have any of the things I had been told I needed to have organized and I was counting on the weekend to get it together. We had a contractor renovating the house we had just moved into and the baby room was far from ready for a baby. It had floor-to-ceiling boxes and Target and Ikea furniture to be assembled. I really needed that weekend.

Fast forward to Monday night when we headed to the hospital. We were running behind and failed to grab food as we headed to the birth of our child. We inaccurately believed that once I had checked in we would have time for Geoff to run to a burrito place in the Mission while whatever drug they would give me to induce would take effect.

Nope!

First, we were late for our 8:00 pm appointment (what, they're going to give our reservation away?) and once checked in, the nurse informed me that I wouldn't be able to eat anything in the event I had to be given medication. So food was off the table for me...and by extension, Geoff. It was going to be a hungry night.

I changed into my hospital gown and the nurse started querying me about my medical history and this pregnancy.

"Wow. Two cancers in one year. I sure hope you had an egg donor because it's not like you'd want to pass your DNA on to a child!"

Um. Ouch...but probably right.

"Any cramping or starting of labor?" Nope!

The nurse brought in a very friendly female doctor a little older than me to perform a sonogram, which is when they found the baby still in breech position.

"Didn't you have a version?"

"Yup. In week 38, but it flipped back. And flipped again. It is a very flippy baby."

"I can't believe they let you go home with a breech baby. They should have admitted you last week. Let me grab another doctor and let's see if we can flip it again."

For the next 30 minutes two medium-sized female doctors pushed and pulled at my belly. This time it was much more uncomfortable because the baby was simply bigger and there was less room for the flipping. So the first doctor recommended they give me an epidural (good thing I hadn't eaten) and they would bring in another, larger doctor to help out.

I was wheeled into an operating room and Geoff was asked to wait outside while they gave me the epidural. As a child, my biologist mother had told me about epidurals previously and how they worked. I was obsessed with the super rare instances where epidurals go horribly wrong and people end up with blinding headaches or worse. So while I was thrilled to reduce my discomfort, I was also not super excited about the whole epidural thing.

And since the medical center is a teaching hospital, I had a resident giving me my epidural. *Sigh*. And yes, it took six tries before the epidural went in right. Then, once it was in, they laid me down and started pumping stuff into me.

The world suddenly got super cold and I felt like I was in another room. I could hear the voices around me but they seemed far away and like I was sinking down to the bottom of a very cold lake. And the nausea was back. Icky. I tried to explain this to the anesthesiologist from a million miles away as I sank deeper down. He checked my blood pressure and apparently I had taken some kind of weird dip. He adjusted some stuff and I came back to the land of the living.

At this point, Geoff was allowed back in the room. Poor guy. He had been standing outside that whole time wondering if he had been forgotten in the excitement of doctors preparing to get medieval on me—or worse, that there was suddenly a problem. But no problem... except that once the larger doctors were assembled, they could *not* get that baby to turn either. No matter how hard they pushed. I could feel the operating table moving back and forth as they pulled on that baby, but I couldn't feel the discomfort I had felt previously (thank *God*).

"Well, it doesn't look like this baby is going to move. Our options now are that we do a cesarean section or we wait until morning when we can find a doctor who can deliver breech babies," said the female doctor.

"What's best for the baby?" I asked.

"Cesarean," she reported.

"Then let's have a baby," I said and the team got to work.

At 12:01am on April 26, 2016, Rory Elizabeth McDonald was born.

LIFE WITH BABY

My friends who have multiple children have told me that the first child is the most challenging and the second child is easier to parent, in part, because the parents are more relaxed. Geoff and I therefore resolved to pretend like Rory was our second child. We would be relaxed. We wouldn't freak out. She would pick up on our zen approach to parenting and by extension, she would be a zen baby. We still have some moments of un-zen, but the whole baby-in-your-late-forties thing has been okay. Granted, most of my high school friends were sending their children off to college while mine was still in diapers—but the whole experience has been *awesome*.

Not surprisingly, the biggest challenge of parenting for Geoff and me has been how to adjust to the new work/life construct. Previously, either of us could leave for work as early—or work as late—as was required. Working on our laptops at night while watching the news was common and accepted by both of us. However, with this new person in our lives all of that had to be renegotiated—with our managers, with one another, and with ourselves.

We had each observed friends making those trade-offs when they had a child, and I think somehow you understand when it is someone else. For each of us, the toughest negotiation was the one we each had with our own sense of ourselves. We thought of ourselves as highly dependable workers. It was difficult when projects couldn't be completed as quickly because the unlimited nighttime work hours no longer existed now that we had Rory. It's a major shift in your self-image and hard to adjust to when you don't feel quite ready to sideline your career—to stop pushing for that next promotion. Add to it commutes that are 75-90 minutes each way on a good day, and there was a lot of stress in the McDonald household.

Wow, I thought. We made it through prior work stresses, infertility issues, cancer (twice!), the death of my father, buying a house, a house renovation, my pregnancy, and each time I felt like we were stronger as a couple for the difficult experience. But wow, juggling full-time jobs and a baby—and we even had full-time help with our nanny, Rossy—we each felt like we were sacrificing our careers and barely hanging on.

I TURN 50

Sensing we needed some time away, Geoff asked that we both take the day off for my birthday, and we drove up to Napa for the day. Geoff had arranged a spa day for us both at the Carneros Inn, which included access to one of their bungalows so we could relax and have a "home" for the day.

It felt like the first time in a long time that we had been just the two of us in the car, talking. We probably spent the majority of the time on the drive up discussing the latest Rory development, but at some point I started telling Geoff about the nerve pain I was having on the left side of my jaw, near my ear. It was really close to where I had been radiated for the adenoid cystic carcinoma five years earlier. The pain was kind of like a sunburn feeling and it would get so intense sometimes that I found myself waking up in the night. I mused aloud that maybe what I was experiencing was "radiation recall" from the radiation I received five years ago.

"Huh. When's your next appointment with Dr. HeadNeck?" he asked.

"I generally set up time with him in early January," I said.

"I'd call him now. In fact, why don't you call him *right now* before we get to Carneros."

I called and described the pain to the nurse on the line. I told her I'd be coming to see the doctor in January, so maybe we should just wait until then? The nurse told me she'd call back once she had spoken with Dr. HeadNeck and she did just as we were pulling into Carneros.

"He'd like to see you this week. Can you come in tomorrow?" she asked.

From my year of treatment, I knew Dr. HeadNeck's schedule was a crazy, packed one that filled up weeks in advance. I knew that for him to ask to see me that week—the next day—was not a good sign. I didn't feel like I could take a day off without notice, so I negotiated for an appointment for the following week.

Everything around me started to slow down as I let my conversation with the nurse sink in. Even before seeing the doctor and running any tests (hadn't I just had a clean MRI in January?) I began to play out the what-ifs. What if I was part of the statistics of people who have a recurrence after five years? What if the cancer was more aggressive this time? What if it had moved up my nerve into my ears, into my eyes, into my brain? What if the tumor was inoperable this time? What if they've done all the radiation they can do on me?

I did my best to focus on being in the moment with Geoff at the spa. I pushed away the what-ifs and focused on the what-is. We were the only ones in the restaurant and had rosé wine with lunch. We were massaged. We spent time in the hot tub. We meandered to our dinner reservations. I had the perfect birthday ("for now," I whispered to myself). *Was this my last birthday?* I asked myself fearfully.

When I met with Dr. HeadNeck the following week, I described to him my symptoms and asked about radiation recall five years out.

"No. We don't see that. What you're describing sounds like it may be progression of the disease, but before we jump to that conclusion, I'd like to run some tests. When was your last head and neck MRI?"

"January of this year. I always get it in January and then meet with you."

"Sarah, your chart shows your last MRI was in June of 2016, just after you had the baby, and I don't think we've seen you since then."

Oh my God. Had I allowed myself to be so distracted by the baby that I had stopped managing my own care? How could I have forgotten to get my annual MRI? In doing so, had we lost valuable months in the treatment of the progression of this disease? And if I had forgotten to schedule the MRI or the appointment with Dr. HeadNeck, why hadn't they picked that up and called me to schedule one or both of those things?

"I don't know. I don't like that we seemed to have missed it too, but let's get an MRI and a CT scan done immediately—and we'll meet again as soon as the results are in. We'll decide our next steps from there," said Dr. HeadNeck very calmly and reasonably.

I searched Dr. HeadNeck's eyes to see if I was overreacting to what I thought he was saying—that my cancer might be back, that it may have progressed—but I only saw him looking very seriously back at me. I thanked him and walked zombie-like from the room.

For three weeks, I went through the motions of going to work. I drove to and from the office, I went to meetings, I suppose I did work. But most of the day I heard the familiar drumbeat of "I have cancer, I have cancer, I have cancer" again in my head. During those three weeks I had both the MRI and the CT scan and waited for the results.

We hosted Thanksgiving dinner with Geoff's parents visiting from Connecticut and my whole extended and immediate family who drove up from Southern California. I took two long hikes with my brother and sister-in-law, and the whole time I had my cancer-progression-confession on the tip of my tongue—wanting so much to share with them the fear I was feeling, but also not wanting to bring them into the stress of the unknown as we had done the first time. Before we knew what we were dealing with. Before we knew my prognosis. So I remained quiet and listened to the voice inside my head that was chanting the cancer earworm.

As I sat on the couch each night and battled with myself not to allow my fear to take hold of me, I was amazed how I had forgotten the visceral physical manifestations of fear. I had forgotten the you-just-rode-a roller-coaster abyss in my stomach. The tingling in my armpits extending out into my arms from the fight-or-flight feeling. The exhaustion.

How had I forgotten all of this in five short years? What was the great mistake I had made that suddenly thrust me back into this hell? Had I become careless? Ungrateful? Without the weekly pace of appointments and tests, had I relaxed? Had I forgotten that with a cancer diagnosis, I could never, ever stop being vigilant about my health? Like all living beings, had I started to believe again in my own immortality?

So convinced was I that my cancer had progressed, I proactively met with Tom, the head of HR for eBay North America, to alert him of my likely need for a medical leave of absence. I asked that he keep this to himself until I received the tests back. I left his office shell-shocked that I was going through all of this again.

I received a notice in my online medical chart that my tests were in. Thankfully, I was working from home that day and could read them in private between conference calls.

The tests. Came. Back. Negative.

No cancer. No progression of disease.

I read over the results at least five times to make sure I was reading them correctly. I called Geoff and read them to him. Then I read them again.

I emailed Dr. HeadNeck and asked for his interpretation of the results. Within two hours I had a message back from him in my inbox.

"There is no indication of malignancy. The tests came back negative. I don't know what it is that you're experiencing, but it's not a malignancy that's causing it. This is not the progression of your disease."

And with that, I was back in the land of the living again.

I drove down to eBay the next day and walked past Tom's office. He made eye contact with me and nodded. He found me as soon as his meeting finished.

"The tests came back negative. I don't have cancer."

Tom looked at me and *he* started crying.

CHAPTER EIGHTEEN

WE MUST DO WHAT IS
IN OUR HEARTS

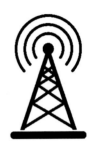

"Our time here is precious. And short. So we must do what is in our hearts."

My new friend Shawn (diagnosed with adenoid cystic carcinoma in 2017) said this to me on the phone this morning as I sat down to write this final chapter. Shawn is closer to her year of treatments than I am. She still retains the Buddha-like wisdom that comes with sitting with a cancer diagnosis. She looks at the world with the understanding that her time here is brief. There is no time to waste when your time is short. You quickly focus only on what is most important to you and cut out everything extraneous. Everything else is noise.

During the three weeks I believed I was having a recurrence, I thought a lot about whether I would have regrets if the cancer had in fact returned and /or had spread. What kept bubbling up for me is the deep regret I would have if I didn't finish writing the book I wanted to write about having cancer. I told Geoff I wanted to quit work for a year to write it. And to his credit, Geoff said, "Yes. If you need to do it – Do It." I checked in with both Kristin and Devin who generously suggested a year-long leave of absence from eBay rather than quitting. "At the end of a year of writing you'll know if that's the path you want to go down," Devin wisely told me over drinks.

I decided to take time off to write a book.
I started writing this book during my year of cancer treatments and then along the way Life Happened and it took me ten years to finish it. Writing a memoir feels arrogant and self-absorbed – even when you have the best of intentions to do it to help others. I hoped my stories could be funny and revealing and help others who find themselves facing cancer feel less alone. Writing my stories down helped me become more reflective; it has helped me better understand who I am, post-cancer.

Who am I, post-cancer? How do I live my life differently? What were the epiphanies I had living through the most frightening year of my life? I get these questions a lot. Here's what I think:

Life is precious and short.

Shawn's quote is simply beautiful and absolutely the way I try to live my life now. In the early days of diagnosis—when my prognosis was unclear and I didn't know if I would be alive by year end—all I wanted, to the core of my being, was to spend more time with Geoff, my family, and my closest friends. I kept thinking: I just want more time. So now that I have been granted more time, I want to ensure I'm focused on the things that will make me happiest during my time here. I actively work to deepen my relationships with my essential people. I text or call, I write handwritten notes, I schedule coffee or wine and hikes, I plan dinner parties and weekends away with those essential people.

We must do what is in our hearts.

This second part of Shawn's quote reminds me that we must be true to what is in our hearts – what we are called to do by our souls. I want to be someone who leaves this life having done the things I wanted to do. So – I have created personal goals for myself which are effectively my no-regrets/bucket list. These help me to keep promises to myself so that if the cancer comes back tomorrow, I will have lived my life as fully as possible. Doing what was in my heart meant taking a year+ off to write a book about my cancer experience with the aspiration that it is both helpful and hopeful.

There was some good that came out of my year of cancer.

I know it is controversial to say – but my year of cancer wasn't *all bad*. Yes, I get that since my outcome was good (I lived), that perhaps colors my evaluation of the year. I am sure it does. But I think it is also because *good stuff did happen* that year that impacts the way I live now. Here are some of the big things I changed, post-cancer:

I chose my life over my work
The work I did was central to my identity for decades. I loved what I did and I think I was good at it. And it is not that the work I do is no longer important to me—it is. It is simply a lower priority when compared to the *people* in my life. And it was for that reason that after my leave of absence to write a book, I made the extremely difficult decision to leave eBay. At its essence, eBay's mission is to enable economic opportunity for all. That mission is/was good and true and worth working for the 14 years I worked at eBay. I believed that mission to the core of my being. And my God I felt I owed so much to the good people of eBay for their (AMAZING!) support of me during my year of cancer! But after Geoff and I moved to Marin County, my commute became two hours each way on a good day. It was simply too much time out of my day and too far from the people I loved most...so I quit. I chose my life over my work. In the work/life balance conundrum, I continue to clearly and intentionally choose my life.

I committed to saying what is in my heart.
For most of my life, I have been described as "outspoken." I have said what is on my mind. What I haven't always done is said what is in my

heart. This sometimes takes a tremendous amount of courage depending on what it is I have needed to say and to whom. But I now reason that if my time is short, I want to ensure I am not leaving things unsaid. This means I say aloud when my feelings are hurt, even if it is embarrassing to admit it. This means I challenge people I love dearly when I believe their actions are in conflict with their integrity. This means I have told people I work with (people I work with!) that I love them. It is a more vulnerable way to live but whew – I have found it is a truer way to live.

I decided to stop worrying about Time.
I am a total fangirl of Lin-Manuel Miranda. I have lost count of the number of times Geoff and I have watched *Hamilton* (and *Encanto*, for that matter). Any article that mentions Lin is immediately click-bait for me. He recently shared on Twitter that he was asked, "Why is there always a ticking clock in your shows?" to which he replied, "Because there is always a ticking clock!" Boy did that resonate with me. I lived most of my life with the sound of a distant ticking in my head – aware and haunted by the watches I wore (and collected) to keep on schedule. At the beginning of my year of cancer treatments, I took my watch off. At first it was because I worried I would leave it in the imaging room at Stanford. Better to keep it at home and safe. After a while, I noticed that without a watch I spent less time checking the time. My day became less driven by what time it was. I still had doctors' appointments to get to, but there was less time-related stress in my life. And I liked it. I now live my life without my watch. I figure if my time is short—I shouldn't spend it counting the minutes to my next appointment or deadline; I should spend my life leaning into the adventure of it.

I decided to have a baby.
If my time was short – I wanted to live as intensely and fully as I could. I wanted the experience of being pregnant, of delivering a baby, and of nurturing an infant. In many ways it was a very selfish decision because it centered on the experiences *I* wished to have. I believed the physical and

emotional transformation I would undergo in becoming a mother was something I did not want to miss.

Unquestionably, my cancer experience informed my new perspective on life – but having a child changed that life. Cancer and a child both taught me to be present for the here and now; Don't wish days or weeks away because you are going through a tough time or you are anticipating an exciting event coming up. Be present. Live through it. Experience the challenging and the exciting, the bad and the good. Because there will be a whole lot of good – especially if you look for it.

Having a child also revealed to me that extraordinary moments happen on ordinary days. If I am busy wishing away those ordinary (sometimes boring, sometimes difficult) days – I will miss the extraordinary moments with my girl.

And, because you are a captive audience, I need to tell you three of my favorite extraordinary Rory stories.

Story #1: We are family.
We drove up to Healdsburg on a Saturday to spend the afternoon with the MacPhails – our friends in the wine business. James and Kerry have placed a long, rustic picnic table in the middle of their overgrown garden which sits to the right of their winery. Kerry grabbed opened bottles from the winery for us to sample and we feasted on the picnic spread we had curated. Rory swung in the hammock with Madi, James and Kerry's daughter, who was on Spring break from college. Rory loved having the attention of a "big girl" and when she wasn't focused on Madi – she was playing with their new puppy, Roxy. It was a most excellent day for a six-year-old (and for a 54-year-old too, I might add).

When we got home, Rory cuddled up to me on the couch and whispered to me, "Mommy, I had such a great day – I LOVE our family!" My heart absolutely melted with her words and as I was in the middle of saying just that to her, she stepped back from me, put her arms over her head and shouted, "WE! ARE! THE MACPHAILS!"

I suppressed a giggle and gently told her, "No, sweetheart, we are the McDonalds. The MacPhails are our friends."

"Do you think they'd let us join their family?" she ardently asked.

*   *   *

Story #2: Daddy.
One Saturday while Geoff was sailing, Rory and I decided to bake banana bread. As I gathered ingredients, I realized we didn't have enough butter. When I announced to Rory that we needed to go to the market, she crossed her arms, stomped her foot, and declared, "I'm not going!"

Teasingly I told her, "Well ok – you can stay home alone then!"

"NO, Mommy! Then the police will come and put me in jail!" she screeched, beginning to panic.

Giggling at her reaction, but also realizing I had freaked her out, I put my arms around her and assured her, "No, honey, I'm the one they'd put in jail."

Her tensed little body immediately relaxed as she looked up at me and said, "Well, then at least I guess I'd have Daddy!"

*   *   *

Story #1: Boys.
After eBay, I spent almost two years working as COO at a small start up located in the Presidio Park of San Francisco. During COVID, we all worked remotely and during one of the leadership team meetings I was running, Rory burst into the room and jumped up on my lap. The other executives all kindly said hello to Rory and welcomed her to the meeting.

Ignoring their comments to her – she looked at me and said, "Mommy. Why are they all boys?!"

*   *   *

With Rory, my life is a series of these extraordinary moments that happen on my most ordinary days. I do my best to be present for them, to be grateful for her, and to remember that all of this could have been different.

I am very lucky.
I am lucky because neither of my cancers was aggressive – so we had time to fight them. I am lucky because my work was fully supportive of me taking time off to focus entirely on my cancer treatments. I am lucky I married the right guy.

I cried a whole lot when I was first diagnosed. But I can only remember Geoff crying once and that was when Dr. BreastOnc told us I wasn't going to be able to carry a child. It was then that the current disaster of our lives became overwhelming for him. It was the only time in our cancer journey that I suspect his focus wasn't entirely on ME—and MY health—and how he could support ME. For a moment, he allowed himself to consider his own feelings and the impact this was all having on HIM.

He might lose his wife. He might never have a child.

These are really BIG existential concerns that he swallowed in order to be there entirely for ME most of that year.

I'm not sure I had the capacity to consider him or his feelings during my year of cancer – so absorbed was I in my own experience of it. Lucky for me – Geoff didn't challenge that capacity. He asked almost nothing of me that year. He just kept showing up with me for all of the doctor appointments – iPad in hand to capture the doctor's answers to my questions. He showed up for the chemo infusions – laptop balanced on his knees while the nurses pumped pink chemicals into his wife. He showed up by holding me when I couldn't hold it together and became overwhelmed by the uncertainty of my prognosis.

He just kept showing up.

It was a long year. It still seems unimaginable that I was diagnosed with two cancers concurrently – and that I survived both. It is miracle #1 that I am now "no evidence of disease" for the salivary gland cancer. It is miracle #2 that I am now "no evidence of disease" for the breast cancer. And maybe the biggest miracle is the fact that I was able to carry a child whom we named Rory. One year. Two cancers. And three utterly amazing miracles.

After all, three is the magic number. Yes it is. Yes it is.

POSTSCRIPT

Naive. Arrogant. Optimistic. These are three words that I feel appropriately described me as I sat down to write this book.

I was accustomed to writing strategy proposals at work. Both as a strategy consultant at Accenture and in various roles at eBay, I would be given 2-4 weeks to pull together a high-level list of objectives with clear metrics and goals to be attained, as well as a comprehensive plan for how we would execute this strategy. After you've done a couple of these, you become acquainted with the format of the proposal, you understand how to create a compelling executive summary, and you and the thesaurus spend a lot of time together thinking of different ways to say "execute" (e.g. "drive," "deliver," "complete," "effect," you get the picture). So I thought this whole book-writing thing might not be easy, but (probably) no harder than writing a strategy proposal.

Except that it turns out writing a book *is* hard. Even when you know the story. It is kind of like putting together a 10,000-piece puzzle. Except when you're writing your own book you don't get a picture on the box to guide you. Turns out you have to sit down and negotiate with yourself every day as to what that picture looks like. And then when you think you've got all of the corner pieces and "frame" pieces in place, you realize that the majority of your puzzle is blue sky. Ugh.

I do love writing though—even when it is hard—and writing this book has been a tremendous way to spend a year+. It has given me the time and space to reflect on all that happened the year I was diagnosed with cancer(s), and how it affected me then and has shaped me since.

I kept a blog during my year of cancer treatments to keep family and friends up to speed on what was going on with me both physically and emotionally. It was a terrific way to keep everyone informed while not exhausting me. It was also a helpful exercise for me to express and explain my personal roller coaster to all who wanted to hear. And, in writing this book, it was an invaluable reminder of what that year was.

My initial blog post was probably the hardest because I felt very vulnerable, almost embarrassed, that I was writing to all of these people about one of the most personal topics I could—my health—and possibly, if things went really sideways, my death. It felt melodramatic to be speaking of matters of life or death, but that is what a cancer diagnosis can be, and I feared I was potentially narrating my own death. So I decided that if my time was limited, I would focus on living as gracefully and fully as I could. Below is the note I sent out to the family and friends who so desperately wanted to help us during that time:

How you can help us.

We need your unconditional love and constant prayers to whatever higher power you believe in. :-) We need you to listen and to discuss this most scary topic with us — but also talk with us about subjects *not* related to cancer as well. We're exhausted from the "all-cancer-all-the-time" channel we've been tuned into. We understand we're going to be living with cancer for the rest of our lives together — but we'd like to focus on the LIVING part of that statement — not the CANCER part of that statement.

I have been very lucky to spend the last ten years *focusing on the living part* – and while my to-do list has expanded – "live" is still at the top of the priority list. But – having completed this book – I have one more bucket list item I can cross off.

May you be well. May you be happy. May you find peace.

Sarah

FREE GIFTS FROM SARAH!

What? You say you want MORE? Well, why didn't you say so....

I have some lists of recommendations I would love to offer you for FREE. These are my opinions based upon my experience as a cancer patient. I hope they are helpful to you, my kind reader:

- 10 things to do when you receive a cancer diagnosis
- 10 things to do for someone you love who has received a cancer diagnosis
- 5 things not to say to someone diagnosed with cancer (and what to say instead)

Go to www.TheCancerChannelBook.com/freegifts to download any of these lists. In exchange, I will ask for your email address so that I can (very occasionally) email you about what I'm doing and/or what I'm writing. Of course, if I become overly enthusiastic about the emailing, you can unsubscribe at any time. I want you to feel supported – not spammed.

Sarah

THANK YOUS

I owe a whole lot of thank you to a whole lot of people.

Life Savers.
Many people saved my life in 2012.

Doctors and Nurses. Most obviously were the medical team at Stanford who were so reassuringly competent in their knowledge of cancer and how it can be treated that I relaxed and trusted these strangers with my life. (I'm looking at you, Melinda and Jessica.)

Family and Friends. The kindness, patience, and prayer extended to me in the darkest moments of my humanity by those I know and hold most dear was humbling. Thank you is not enough, but it is what I have – thankfulness and gratitude.

This book was a big old project for me and I am so very grateful for all of the counsel and support I received as I tried to bring this book to publication.

Readers.
I had the benefit of many supportive readers including **Alan Le, Amy Hansell, Ann Corbett, Chris Loder, Deb Olshefski, Geordie**

McDonald, **Ginger Miller, Jennifer Russell, Karen Snell, Kristin Yetto, LeAyn Dillon, Lyra Olson, Mara Lowry, Sarvenaz Madi, Susan Ford, Susan Meinders, Theresa Fox, Tripti Mahendra, Ulrike Steinbach,** and, of course, **Geoff McDonald**. Thank you for the encouragement you gave, as well as the gentle suggestions you offered. So many of you shaped this book.

Book Cover Designer.

Thank you to **Tiffany Grisham** who is both artist and family. Thank you for your openness to learning this stuff with me and for your bubbly enthusiasm for my stories and this project.

Editors.

Shane Tepper and **Catherine Reilly** served as my initial editors. Catherine (who volunteered to do this!) especially saw the many shitty first drafts. Shane was particularly patient with my reflexive need to double space after every. damned. period. Thank you, both.

Nanette Levin served as my final editor – catching the lapses and repetition I feared lurked in the manuscript – while all the while helping me believe that this was worth finishing. Thank you for pushing me to make it better.

Self-publishing guru.

Diana Needham was my project manager / book sherpa (helping to get me over the summit of self-publishing). Thank you for telling me this was an important story to tell and for giving me the roadmap to do just that.

Husband.

Geoff McDonald, thank you for always showing up – then and now. I choose you.

ABOUT THE AUTHOR

Sarah E. McDonald lives in Mill Valley with her husband, Geoff, and daughter, Rory. Sarah has spent the majority of her 30-year career in the technology industry, 14 years of which were at eBay. Sarah received her MBA from Cornell University and her BA from Occidental College. Beyond cancer, Sarah is interested in all things people-related – especially when paired with food, wine, the outdoors, and/or music. *The Cancer Channel* is her first book.

2012   2022

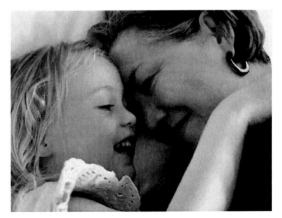

Photo credit:
Renee Boccasile

Photo credit:
Geoff McDonald

Made in United States
North Haven, CT
05 December 2022

27921945R10135